Methods and Designs for Outcomes Research

Methods and Designs for Outcomes Research

Elinor C. G. Chumney, Ph.D.
   Assistant Professor
   Department of Pharmacy and Clinical Sciences
   South Carolina College of Pharmacy
   Charleston, South Carolina

Kit N. Simpson, Dr.P.H.
   Professor and Chair
   College of Health Professions
   Department of Health Administration and Policy
   Medical University of South Carolina
   Charleston, South Carolina

For more than 60 years, ASHP has helped pharmacists who practice in hospitals and health systems improve medication use and enhance patient safety. The Society's 30,000 members include pharmacists and pharmacy technicians who practice in inpatient, outpatient, home-care, and long-term-care settings, as well as pharmacy students. For more information about the wide array of ASHP activities and the many ways in which pharmacists help people make the best use of medicines, visit ASHP's Web site, www.ashp.org, or its consumer Web site, www.SafeMedication.com.

Any correspondence regarding this publication should be sent to the publisher, American Society of Health-System Pharmacists, 7272 Wisconsin Avenue, Bethesda, MD, 20814, attn: Special Publishing. Produced in conjunction with the ASHP Publications Production Center.

The information presented herein reflects the opinions of the contributors and reviewers. It should not be interpreted as an official policy of ASHP or as an endorsement of any product.

Drug information and its applications are constantly evolving because of ongoing research and clinical experience and are often subject to professional judgment and interpretation by the practitioner and to the uniqueness of a clinical situation. The authors and ASHP have made every effort to ensure the accuracy and completeness of the information presented in this book. However, the reader is advised that the publisher, authors, editors, and reviewers cannot be responsible for the continued currency of the information, for any errors or omissions, and/or for any consequences arising from the use of the information in the clinical setting.

The reader is cautioned that ASHP makes no representation, guarantee, or warranty, express or implied, that the use of the information contained in this book will prevent problems with insurers and will bear no responsibility or liability for the results or consequences of its use.

Acquisitions Editor: *Hal Pollard*
Editorial Project Manager: *Dana A. Battaglia*
Senior Project Editor: *Bill Fogle*
Composition: *Carol A. Barrer*
Cover and page design: *Armen Kojoyian*

ISBN: 1-58528-111-5

Dedication

To Wade, Morgan, Mary, and my parents for their love and understanding. E.C.G.C.

To Annie and Chris for their patience and support. K.N.S.

Furthermore, we jointly dedicate this book to our colleagues and students from whom we continue to learn so much.

Table of Contents

Section One: Study Design

Chapter 1
Introduction to Study Design   3
Elinor C. G. Chumney, Ph.D.

Chapter 2
Measuring Disease and Outcome Frequency   5
Richard M. Schulz, Ph.D.

Chapter 3
Ecologic Analysis   23
Elinor C. G. Chumney, Ph.D.

Chapter 4
Epidemiologic Study Designs   29
Vicki M. Young, Ph.D., R.Ph, Pamela J. Mazyck, Pharm.D., Richard M. Schulz, Ph.D.

Chapter 5
Randomized Clinical Trials   45
Patrick D. Mauldin, Ph.D., and Jean Nappi, Pharm.D., FCCP, BCPS

Chapter 6
Meta-Analysis   57
Anne P. Spencer, Pharm.D.

Section Two: Descriptive Statistics and Univariate Analysis

Section Three: Regression Analysis

Section Four: Integrative Models

Section Five: Pharmacoeconomic Analysis

Acknowledgments

We would like to acknowledge the tremendous contribution of our coauthors, who are all experts in their respective areas. Without their responsiveness to the learning needs of health professional students, we never would have accomplished the writing of this book. It has truly been a collaborative effort.

Special thanks go to our Editorial Project Manager, Dana Battaglia, our Senior Project Editor, Bill Fogle, and our Layout Artist, Carol A. Barrer, for all their help in this endeavor.

It is also important to acknowledge the contribution of Dr. John Bosso, Chairman of the Department of Pharmacy and Clinical Sciences in the South Carolina College of Pharmacy. Over the years, he has provided a supportive environment and permitted us to find the time and resources necessary to complete this text. We also wish to thank D'Jaris Whipper-Lewis and Helen Gary for their invaluable assistance.

Finally, we would like to express our appreciation to the thorough and professional reviewers, anonymous to us, whose careful consideration contributed greatly to the development of this book.

Preface

Our experiences in designing and teaching outcomes research courses in colleges of pharmacy and health professions over the last 7 years have convinced us of the pressing need for a textbook to cover this broad research area. The field of outcomes research includes equal measures of pharmacoepidemiology, statistics, and pharmacoeconomics. Although there are numerous texts devoted to one or the other, there has not yet been a book that could satisfactorily and coherently synthesize the material for our students.

As we pulled the textbook together, we approached leaders within each academic discipline and asked them to author chapters specific to their field of interest. The result is a broad overview of the field of outcomes research.

The book is designed primarily for graduate students in health-related degree programs, including pharmacy, medicine, nursing, and health administration. It will introduce clinical professionals and students to common statistical methods and study designs used in pharmacoepidemiology and outcomes research, as well as to issues related to the measurement, analysis, and interpretation of results of clinical trials and outcomes studies. In crafting this textbook, we were especially concerned with conveying the tools for the appropriate interpretation of various analyses to best guide future practice decisions. We focused our efforts on explanations with words rather than complex mathematical formulas, using health care databases and examples to illustrate important concepts.

Section 1 aims to teach the reader to understand the strengths and limitations of controlled trials, observational, quasi-experimental, and epidemiological designs. Richard Schulz, Ph.D., begins this section by covering measurements of disease and outcome frequency. After an intermediate chapter on ecologic analysis (by Chumney), he co-authored a second chapter on case-control and cohort studies with Vicki Young, Ph.D., and Pamela Mazyck, Pharm.D., Patrick Mauldin, Ph.D., and Jean Nappi, Pharm.D., co-authored the chapter on randomized clinical trials, considered to be the gold standard of epidemiologic study designs. Anne P. Spencer, Pharm.D., completes this section with a chapter on meta-analyses, which allow researchers to combine the results of several smaller studies into a more powerful assessment of effect.

Nannette Berenson, Pharm.D., provides a comprehensive overview of statistics in chapter 7, including descriptive statistics, hypothesis testing, and measures of association.

Section 3 expands on statistical analysis by focusing on regression analyses; to facilitate comparisons within this section, all of the chapters based their examples on the same database. Richard Lindrooth, Ph.D., and Libby Dismuke, Ph.D., co-authored the chapter on ordinary least squares (OLS) regression. Edward Norton, Ph.D., and Sally Stearns, Ph.D., co-authored the chapter on logistic regression. The final chapter of this section focuses on sample selection models.

Decision trees and Markov models are covered in Chapter 11. This chapter explores the contribution of integrative modeling studies used to estimate outcomes for specific patient groups in the short and long term.

Section 5 covers pharmacoeconomic analyses. Gene Reeder, Ph.D., reviews cost-effectiveness analysis (CEA). After a chapter on cost-utility analysis (CUA), Jo Mauskopf, Ph.D., Richard Berzon, Ph.D., and Francis S. Lobo, Ph.D., expand on these issues with chapters on measuring utilities and measuring health-related quality of life. David Bradford, Ph.D., concludes this section with a chapter on cost benefit analysis (CBA). Finally, the Appendix summarizes how to critically read published papers that incorporate patient outcome and cost measures.

We hope our readers enjoy and learn from this book, and we wish them all the best in their pursuits related to outcomes research.

Elinor C. G. Chumney
Kit N. Simpson
September, 2005

Contributors

Nannette M. Berensen, Pharm.D., BCPS
Associate Professor
Department of Pharmacy and Clinical Sciences
Coordinator,
Drug Information Services
South Carolina College of Pharmacy
Charleston, South Carolina

Richard A. Berzon, Ph.D.
HIV/AIDS Technical Advisor
U.S. Agency for International Development
Bureau for Global Health, Office of HIV/AIDS
Washington, DC

David Bradford, Ph.D.
Professor and Director
Center for Health Economic and Policy Studies
Medical University of South Carolina
College of Health Professions
Department of Health Administration and Policy
Charleston, South Carolina

Elinor C. G. Chumney, Ph.D.
Assistant Professor
Department of Pharmacy and Clinical Sciences
South Carolina College of Pharmacy
Charleston, South Carolina

Clara E. Dismuke, Ph.D.
Assistant Professor
Center for Health Economic and Policy Studies
Medical University of South Carolina
College of Health Professions
Department of Health Administration and Policy
Charleston, South Carolina

Richard C. Lindrooth, Ph.D.
Associate Professor
Center for Health Economics and Policy
Department of Health Administration and Policy
College of Health Professions
Medical University of South Carolina
Charleston, South Carolina

Francis S. Lobo, Ph.D.
Assistant Director
Health Economics and Outcomes Research
Novartis Pharmaceuticals Corporation
East Hanover, New Jersey

Patrick D. Mauldin, Ph.D.
Associate Professor
Department of Pharmacy and Clinical Sciences
South Carolina College of Pharmacy
Charleston, South Carolina

Josephine Mauskopf, Ph.D.
Vice President
Health Economics
RTI Health Solutions
Research Triangle Park, North Carolina

Pamela J. Mazyck, Pharm.D.
Clinical Pharmacist
Medical University of South Carolina
Charleston, South Carolina

Jean Nappi, Pharm.D., FCCP, BCPS
Professor
Department of Pharmacy and Clinical Sciences
South Carolina College of Pharmacy
Charleston, South Carolina

Edward C. Norton, Ph.D.
Professor
University of North Carolina at Chapel Hill
Department of Health Administration and Policy
Chapel Hill, North Carolina

Claiborne E. Reeder, R.Ph., Ph.D.
Professor of Pharmacoeconomics
South Carolina College of Pharmacy
Columbia, South Carolina

Richard M. Schulz, Ph.D.
Professor of Health Outcomes Science
South Carolina College of Pharmacy
Columbia, South Carolina

Kit N. Simpson, Dr.P.H.
Professor and Chair
College of Health Professions
Department of Health Administration and Policy
Medical University of South Carolina
Charleston, South Carolina

Anne P. Spencer, Pharm.D.
Associate Professor
South Carolina College of Pharmacy
Department of Pharmacy and Clinical Sciences
Charleston, South Carolina

Sally C. Stearns, Ph.D.
Associate Professor
University of North Carolina at Chapel Hill
Department of Health Policy and Administration
Chapel Hill, North Carolina

Vicki M. Young, Ph.D., R.Ph.
EXCEED Program Fellow
Department of Pharmacy and Clinical Sciences
College of Pharmacy
Medical University of South Carolina
Charleston, South Carolina

Reviewers

Arjun P. Dutta, Ph.D.

J. Russell May, Pharm.D., FASHP

Linda S. Tyler, Pharm.D.

Lee Vermeulen, R.Ph., M.S.

Section One

Study Design

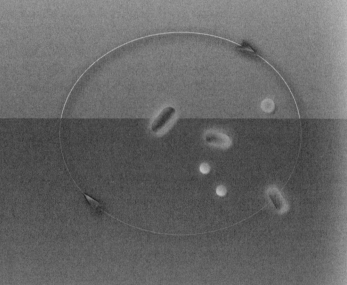

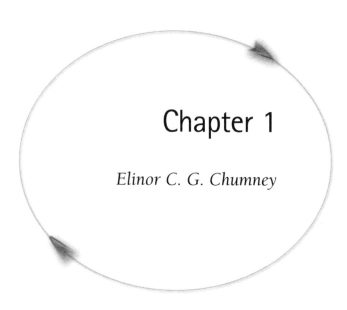

Chapter 1

Elinor C. G. Chumney

Introduction to Study Design

The science of medical care is advanced through research, and we are consumers of that research, both in the classroom and later in providing care for our own patients. This section provides an overview of epidemiologic concepts and study designs to facilitate a better understanding of this vast and productive field of research. Epidemiology is based on the fundamental assumptions that disease does not occur at random, and that both causal and preventive factors can be identified through a systematic investigation of different groups.[1] These investigations, predicated on accurate measurements of disease and outcome frequencies, involve an array of study designs, each with their own unique advantages and limitations.

Knowledge of both the frequency and distribution of a disease is necessary to understand, formulate, and test hypotheses about its determinants, whether causal or preventive. These measurements of disease and outcome frequency, including incidence, prevalence, and mortality rates, are discussed in Chapter 2.

The chapters on study designs are presented in order of the ascending rigor of their design. We begin with a chapter on ecologic analyses (Chapter 3), which involve comparisons of groups and are especially well-suited to exploring relationships between a disease and its potential causes. Typically, the groups are derived from geographically defined areas, such as nations, states, or counties, and the analyses are based on existing data from these populations.

In contrast, case-control, cohort, and randomized clinical trials all focus on comparisons of individuals. Information for these analyses is often gathered through individual interviews, direct observation, or medical records, and is specific for each person included in the study. These approaches are more labor-intensive and expensive, but the pay-off is that they allow researchers to predict individual risk or odds.

Case-control and cohort analyses are observational study designs and are discussed in Chapter 4. Under a case-control study, subjects are selected based on whether they do (cases) or do not (controls) have the disease under investigation. The two groups are then compared based on their respective history of exposures. Case-control analyses tend to be less expensive and less time-consuming than cohort or randomized clinical trials.

Under a cohort study, subjects are selected based on whether or not they were exposed to a suspected risk factor for a disease. At the time exposure status is defined, potential subjects must be free from the disease under investigation. Eligible participants are then followed over a period of time to capture the number of subjects in both groups who develop the disease. Since cohort studies often involve following a large number of subjects for a long time period, they tend to be more time-consuming and expensive than case-control studies.

As discussed in Chapter 5, a randomized clinical trial (RCT) is the most rigorous study design. Patients are assigned to a particular treatment based on chance and are then monitored for a period of time to determine their disease experience.

Finally, we conclude this section with a chapter on meta-analyses (Chapter 6), statistical analyses of a collection of studies. They allow researchers to combine data from a number of previously conducted studies of the same subject to obtain an overall estimate of effect. However, it is important to remember that the quality and usefulness of any meta-analysis is dependent on the quality and comparability of the individual studies included therein.

Reference

1. Hennekens CH, Buring JE. *Epidemiology in Medicine*. Boston: Little, Brown, and Company; 1987.

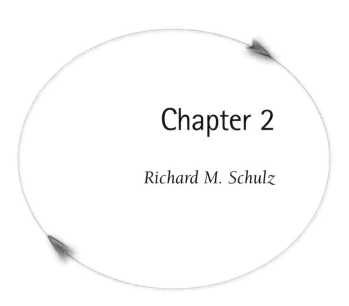

Chapter 2

Richard M. Schulz

Measuring Disease and Outcome Frequency

Introduction

Textbooks that attempt to bring clarity to the scientific process are frequently met with suspicion by students, and frequently with good cause. Everyone has encountered texts in which knowing and understanding the material appears to be a prerequisite for understanding the book—a classic academic Catch-22. Authors' dependence on scientific notation and arcane formulas only adds to the student's dilemma. In effect, students are asked to learn new material by using and applying information and skills they have not mastered.

The solution to this problem may be surprising. The solution is not found in eliminating the notations or formulas, because they serve an important and useful role. Rather, the solution is recognizing that the fundamental building block of measuring disease and outcome frequency has already been mastered. That building block is counting. Pop culture is replete with references to counting and its importance in understanding and interpreting the world. For the young at heart, Sesame Street's character, The Count, used numbers and counting to make sense of the physical world. For the more erudite, the current television show, "Numbers," seeks to explain human behavior as an expression of mathematical relationships. The issue is given a historical referent by the noted 19th century physicist James Maxwell, who stated "We owe all great advances in knowledge to those who endeavor to find out how much there is of anything." So, while this chapter contains new material, including formulas that will be unfamiliar and challenging, the skill necessary to understand the content of the chapter has already been mastered. To paraphrase the title of Robert Fulghum's signature work, "All You Really Need to Know about Measuring Disease and Outcome Frequency You Learned in Kindergarten."

Counting is equally important to the clinician caring for an individual patient as to the epidemiologist or health service administrator attempting to understand the health and health care needs of populations. Physicians, nurses, and pharmacists assess the presence and/or severity of a medical condition by determining values of parameters relevant to the condition, and comparing the values to standards. Clinicians caring for individuals suspected of having contracted HIV will measure viral load and CD4 cell counts to make a diagnosis, determine severity, or judge the success of therapy. Health care professionals treating asthma patients will count the number of nighttime awakenings due to asthma symptoms, or measure the change in symptom-free days to assess the effectiveness of a particular intervention. Pharmacists will count the number of days beyond expected refill date to assess the degree to which a patient has been adherent to a prescribed treatment regimen. At a population level, epidemiologists need to count the number of new cases of a particular medical condition to determine if it is increasing in the population, and, therefore, becoming a growing health care problem. Epidemiologists and health planners need to assess disease trends to better plan for the care required by ever-larger numbers of patients. Regardless of whether the focus is the individual patient or the population, improved diagnosis, treatment, and planning is dependent on an unambiguous way of counting and a systematic way of reporting and interpreting the results.

The process of counting results in the clinician or scientist knowing the number of events that occur, or the number of people who have had an event. This is especially applicable in outcomes research, where the number of side effects, hospitalizations, emergency department visits, or even deaths, is the outcome of interest. Unfortunately, while the simplicity of counting events is compelling, it offers only a partial, and sometimes incorrect, interpretation of the data.

The following example illustrates this point (Table 2.1). A hospital pharmacy director plans to initiate a quality improvement program to address the growing number of medication errors detected. In advance of the program, she conducts a needs assessment to determine the service or floors most in need of the intervention. One medical service has a clinical pharmacist working full time, while the other medical service does not. Medication errors are recorded over a 1-month period using a standard data collection instrument. To her surprise, the service with clinical pharmacist reported 36 medication errors; the service without the clinical pharmacist reported only 20 medication errors during the same period. While there may be many reasons for these results, including the additional vigilance associated with the presence of a clinical pharmacist, a fundamental problem is attributed to the inadequacy of count data. The number of errors must be given some context or perspective to be fully understood. Furthermore, without that context, conclusions drawn from the data may be incorrect. Typically, we provide a context by dividing the number of cases or events by the number that represents the population from which the cases emerged. In other words, knowing the number of errors is meaningful only if the total number of medications dispensed on each service is known. A meaningful comparison in this example, therefore, is the number of errors/total number of medications dispensed in each service during the time period. If the medical service with the clinical pharmacist had 36,000 medication orders dispensed, the proportion of medications dispensed that were errors would by 36/36000 = 0.001 = 0.1%. If the service without a clinical pharmacist had 5000 medication orders dispensed, the proportion of medication dispensed that were errors would be 20/5000 = 0.004 = 0.4%. Even though the absolute number of errors was greater in the service served by a clinical pharmacist, the proportion of medications dispensed that contained an error was four times greater in the service without a clinical pharmacist. Without placing the count data in some perspective, the pharmacy director may have committed resources where they were least needed.

Proportions and Rates

In the example above, count data was made more meaningful by dividing it by a number that represents the whole from which the subset of counts came. Of all medications dispensed (denominator), a certain proportion or percentage contained errors (numerator). In effect, we have created a proportion composed of numerator and denominator. The events recorded in the numerator must also be included in the denominator. The 36 medication orders that resulted in errors reported in the numerator must be a part of the population of medication orders dispensed. A unique feature of proportions is that both numerator and denominator have the same units. By dividing two numbers with the same units, the units cancel, leaving a unitless number. As a result, proportions can be reported as fractions (36/36,000), decimals (0.001) or percentages (0.1%). Proportions can be used to report the percentage of a population with hypertension, the fraction of patients with hyperlipidemia that reaches goal, the percentage of HIV patients who remain adherent to prescribed therapy, etc.

Rates are similar to proportions in that both have numerators and denominators. They differ, however, on several important dimensions. A key distinction between rates and proportions is that while the numerator and denominator of proportions have the same units, in rates they have different units. Another important distinction is that rates have some element of time incorporated in the denominator.

The following example demonstrates both points. Nurses administering intravenous medication deal with infusion rates, i.e., the number of milliliters (mL) of medicine infused per hour. In this example, the numerator is the number of mL of medicine infused. The denominator has different units, namely, time (hour). The result of the division is not a unitless number but rather a number that carries the units along. The nurse who adjusts the infusion rate of the medicine so that the patient receives 100 ml in each hour does not report an infusion rate of "100." Instead, the rate is reported as 100 mL/hour. The rate reports some event (infusion of milliliters of medicine) over a period of time (hour). Rates might also be used to report new cases of asthma per 100,000 people during a year period, or deaths

Table 2.1
Error Count and Proportion in Two Services

	Service with Pharm.D.	Service with no Pharm.D.
Medication orders with errors	36	20
Total number of medication orders	36,000	5,000
Proportion of medication orders with errors	0.1%	0.4%

per 1,000 people over 65 due to influenza during the 1990s. In the example of medication errors, a rate could be constructed by using a denominator with units different than the numerator, and with units that incorporated time. In the previous example about medication errors, one could argue that the appropriate comparison is not the number of errors relative to the total number of medicines dispensed, but rather the number of errors relative to the total number of days that a patient occupied a bed, termed a *patient-day.* If the service with a clinical pharmacist had 100 beds, and, during the 30-day month, half the beds were occupied, then the denominator would be 1500 patient-days (100 beds × 30 days × 0.5 occupancy). The error rate per patient day would be 36 errors/1500 patient-days, or 0.024 errors per patient day, or 2.4 errors per 100 patient days. Often, when the calculated value is a decimal, it is multiplied by some factor of 10 to be better understood. In this example, 0.024 errors per patient day is multiplied by 100 to give a rate of 2.4 errors per 100 patient-days. The value of this rate is that it gives an estimate of the likelihood of an error occurring each day (or each 100 days) a bed is occupied. This type of rate will be discussed further in the section on incidence.

Proportions and rates are mathematical expressions whose interpretation can remain the same although their numerical values may change. The proportion of prescription orders that resulted in errors can be presented as 36/36,000, or 1/1,000, or 0.001, or 0.1%. Although the value of the numbers may change, the interpretation of the proportion (or fraction, or percentage) remains the same. The same is true with rates. The infusion rate may be reported as 100 mL per hour, or 1 L/10 hours. The meaning conveyed by these rates is the same.

Rates and proportions are important but generic mathematical expressions used to convey the frequency or occurrence of event. Caution should be taken regarding these two terms. Inconsistencies can be found in the literature due to failure to adhere to the conventions and nomenclature described above. In addition, problems can arise because the terms of both numerator and denominator are inadequately defined. Following up on the example above, the needs assessment indicated that the service with no clinical pharmacist experienced 20 errors per 5,000 medication orders. In the numerator, were there 20 errors, or 20 patients who experienced an error? If an error was repeated on the same patient, would it be counted once or multiple times. In the denominator, should the most meaningful unit be the number of medication orders dispensed or the number of patients who received medication? These questions indicate the need for clarity with respect to the units of both numerator and denominator for proportions and rates, and the need for caution in comparing proportions and rates across studies.

Incidence and Prevalence

The rates and proportions most often used in epidemiology and outcomes research to assess disease or outcome frequency are broadly termed incidence and prevalence. Incidence is defined as the number of new cases of disease or event that develop in a population of individuals at risk over a specified period of time. Two elements of incidence are critical to understanding its meaning. First, the denominator is made up of people who are at risk for contracting the disease or having the event of interest, i.e., they have the potential to contract the disease or experience the event. If a person cannot have the disease or event during the specified time period, then he or she cannot be counted in the denominator. A study of the incidence of hysterectomy in people aged 50–59 from January 1, 2000, to December 31, 2000, cannot include men in the denominator because men physically are unable to have the procedure, and therefore, are not at risk. Likewise, women who have had hysterectomies prior to this time or age can not be included in the denominator, because they are not at risk to have another during the time under study. Second, the numerator is comprised of people who have *transitioned* from non-case status to case status during the time period under study. All women who have not previously had a hysterectomy and who satisfy the age requirement during the specified time period are counted in the denominator. If a woman has a hysterectomy, she is included not only in the denominator, but in the numerator, as well.

Incidence is considered the frequency with which a disease or event develops within a population at risk that is followed over a specified period of time. As such, it is a reflection of new cases that occur during the time period under study. Incidence can be calculated as a proportion or rate. When incidence is calculated as a proportion, it is called incidence proportion or cumulative incidence or attack rate. When incidence is calculated as a rate, it is called incidence rate or incidence density or instantaneous risk.

Cumulative incidence is calculated as follows:

$$CI = \frac{\text{Number of new cases that develop in population at risk over a specified time}}{\text{Number of persons at risk for developing the condition or disease over a specified time}}$$

Semantic variations of this definition of cumulative risk describe the population in the denominator as those at risk at the beginning of the study period. The assumption made is that those persons identified at the beginning of the study will be followed throughout the study period. For cumulative incidence to be measured directly from a population, the population represented in the denominator must be stable, i.e., there can be no additions or subtractions to the denominator over the specified time. Additions after the beginning of the study period are problematic because the presence or absence of the disease at the beginning of the study period cannot be ascertained retrospectively. There is no assurance that the person belongs in the population at risk. Deletions before the study period ends may occur as a result of not being able to follow the person for the specified time, termed, lost to follow-up. This is problematic because the clinician or researcher has no way of determining if the person transitioned to case status after contact was lost. In either situation, the resultant cumulative incidence would not be a correct reflection of the risk or probability of developing the disease or condition over the specified period of time.

Wong et al.[1] examined the association between microvascular disease and the development of subsequent congestive heart failure in a 7-year cohort study in four U.S. communities. Retinopathy was considered a marker of systemic microvascular disease, and was assessed in the population at the beginning of the study. The 7-year cumulative incidence of congestive heart failure in study participants who had been diagnosed with retinopathy at the early stages of the study was 15.1 percent, while the seven year cumulative incidence of study participants who had no signs of retinopathy was 4.8 percent. Study participants who had documented congestive heart failure prior to the retinal exam were excluded from the study, because they were not at risk of becoming a new case of congestive heart failure.

Incidence Density

Recall that the denominator of cumulative incidence is a number of persons that represent the population from which cases have been drawn. Cumulative incidence assumes that members of that population are at risk for the disease, outcome, or condition throughout the period of observation. Additions and subtractions from this population, as described above, are always a possibility. The measure, incidence density, is calculated in such a way to account for these problems. Incidence density does not require that the population remains unchanged throughout the time period. However, it does require that each person's time at risk, regardless of how long or how short, be accounted for in the denominator. This is accomplished by creating a product term, generally considered *person-time*. Each person contributes a certain amount of time to the denominator that corresponds to the time the person was at risk for the outcome. One person who was followed in a study for 90 days would contribute 90 (1 × 90) person-days to the denominator. Three people who each were followed for 30 days would contribute 90 (3 × 30) person-days to the denominator. This example illustrates two important principles of incidence density. First, a quantitative value of person-time can be arrived at in any number of ways. Each unit of person-time has equal value and contribution to the denominator, regardless of how it was created. Second, because each unit of person-time has equal weight, we can sum each person's time in which he or she was followed to arrive at a total person-time in the denominator. Thus, the calculation for incidence density is as follows:

$$ID = \frac{\text{Number of new cases that develop in population at risk over a specified time}}{\text{Total person-time of observation}}$$

An important distinction between cumulative incidence and incidence density should be apparent, given the previous discussion about rates and proportions. Cumulative incidence has the same units in both numerator and denominator (number of people). Cumulative incidence is a proportion whose division yields a unitless number. Incidence density differs from cumulative incidence in several ways. Although the numerators of the two are the same, i.e., number of new cases, the denominator of an incidence density is person-time. Because the denominator incorporates an element of time, incidence density is a rate.

Caution should be exercised when dealing with incidence density values. In the example above, 90 person-days were contributed to the denominator. This can also be presented as 3 person-months. Let's assume that during this time, 3 cases of disease were recorded. This could be reported as 3 cases/90 person-days, 0.033 case/person-day, 3 cases/3 person-months, or 1 case/person-month. All four designations are equivalent but look very different numerically. The numerical value of incidence density is meaningful only in the context of the units of person-time.

Figure 2.1 demonstrates the calculation of incidence density. Each line represents a person and their case/non-case status over time. An "x" indicates the time a person contracted the disease or had the outcome of interest. It indicates the time the person transitioned from non case-to-case status. The figure could represent the observations within a clinical trial, a field experiment, or a historical cohort in which people were followed from a previous starting point forward in time. In this example, we observed people from January 1, 2004, to December 31, 2004.

At first glance, it appears that the numerator should be 4 because four x's are recorded. However, person A already had the disease or outcome prior to the start of the observation period. Because the definition of incidence requires that new cases only be counted, person A cannot be counted in the numerator. During the January 1—December 31 time period, three new cases were recorded. The numerator of the incidence density calculation is "3." The denominator is the sum of the person-time of observation for people who are at risk to develop the disease or outcome. Again, person A's time cannot be included in the denominator because he or she was not at risk to become a new case. The time contribution of each of the remaining people is as follows: B and I: 6 months, C: 3 months, D: 9 months, E, F, H: 12 months each, G: 11 months, J: 10 months.

$$ID = \frac{\text{Number new cases}}{\text{Total person-time observed}} = \frac{3 \text{ new cases}}{81 \text{ person-months}} = 0.037 \text{ cases/person-month}$$

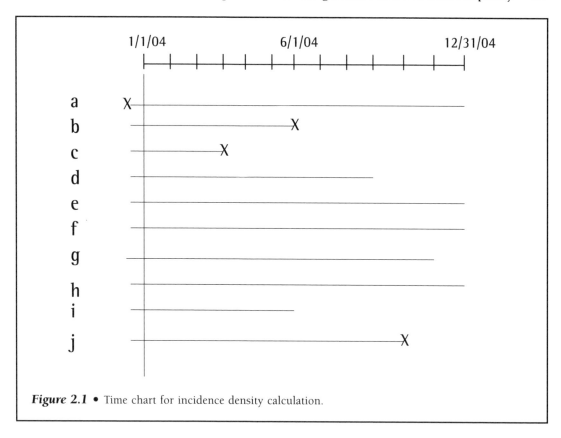

Figure 2.1 • Time chart for incidence density calculation.

Lacoste-Roussillon et al.[2] reported the incidence of serious adverse drug events in general practice, using incidence density as the measure of event frequency. The authors used a stratified random sampling method to identify and select general practitioners to participate in the study. Practitioners then collected information about adverse drug reactions among their patients for a consecutive 5-day period that occurred between March 1 and April 30, 1998. Incidence density of serious adverse events was 10.2 per 1,000 days of practice. Incidence density was the appropriate measure of disease frequency for two reasons: (1) general medical practices entered the study (beginning of 5-day observation period) and left the study (end of 5-day observation period) at various times, and (2) the authors wanted to count the time and adverse event contribution of each general medical practice.

Van Roon et al.[3] prospectively assessed the incidence of withdrawal from leflunomide, a novel compound indicated for rheumatoid arthritis. Patients with rheumatoid arthritis who were prescribed leflunomide in the outpatient setting between January 2000 and June 2002 were included in the study. The outcome of interest was discontinuation or withdrawal from the medicine. Withdrawal was defined as any reported discontinuation for any reason. The authors reported the incidence density for withdrawal was 56.2 per 100 patient-years. As with the study reported above, incidence density was measured so that patient time and withdrawal event could be captured regardless of when the patient was enrolled and when he or she reached an endpoint.

Prevalence

Prevalence is defined as the number of persons in a population who have a particular disease or outcome at a specified time divided by the number of persons in the population at that time. Because the units in both numerator and denominator are the same, prevalence is a proportion. The calculation for prevalence is below:

$$\text{Prevalence} = \frac{\text{Number of cases of disease or outcome at a specified time}}{\text{Number of people in the population at a specified time}}$$

Although the definition and formula for prevalence is similar to those for incidence, there are several important differences. First, prevalence is an assessment of all cases in a population, not just new cases, as with incidence. The calculation of prevalence, therefore, will include both new cases and existing cases. Second, prevalence focuses on the number of cases at a particular point in time, whereas incidence identifies the number of new cases that have developed over some specified period of time. An analogy that may clarify the difference is that prevalence is a snapshot, a still picture, of the disease or outcome in a community; incidence is a video or moving picture of the development of disease or outcome over time. A financial analogy might also be helpful. Prevalence is an individual's or business's balance sheet, including all assets and liabilities at a particular point in time. Incidence is an individual's bank statement or a business's income statement showing the movement of monies through an account over time.

Just as with incidence, there are two measures of prevalence. *Point prevalence* is the number of new and existing cases at a specific point in time divided by the number of people within the population at that time. The other measure of prevalence is called *period prevalence,* in which the time frame is expanded from a particular point in time to some specified period of time. Period prevalence, therefore, is the total number of new and existing cases in a population during a specified period of time divided by some measure of the total population during that period. This denominator may be the population at the midpoint of the time period, or the average of the population at the beginning and the end of the time period. A legitimate use of period prevalence is in determining the frequency of disease or condition that is difficult to determine a date on which a person transitions to a case. An example of such a condition is alcoholism. If point prevalence were used, it would miss the many people who indeed had alcoholism but whose symptoms had not been demonstrated sufficiently to warrant medical diagnosis. The expansion of the time frame allows for a more realistic assessment of the prevalence of the condition in a community.

The astute reader will recognize an inherent problem in the definition of period prevalence, namely, that the expanded time frame suggests that period prevalence captures elements of both point prevalence and incidence. For this reason, period prevalence is infrequently used. When the term prevalence is used without qualifier, it typically refers to point prevalence. However, it is important to recognize those situations in which an expanded time frame is appropriate, and thus the use of period prevalence is warranted.

Prevalence is a measure that reflects the burden of disease. It can be used to determine the amount of resources, whether financial, physical, or human, that will be needed to treat a disease and care for those afflicted. For these reasons, prevalence may be a better measure than incidence for the burden of disease, especially for chronic conditions. Consider the following example. Alzheimer's is a condition associated with progressive cognitive impairment. People with Alzheimer's may live more than 10 years with the condition. As cognitive functioning deteriorates and their ability to perform activities of daily living lessens, these patients require more complex and sophisticated medical and social services. Monies must be allocated for the care of these individuals, physical structures would be needed when the family is unable to provide adequate care, and a broad range of personnel must be in place so that care can be delivered. The number of new cases of Alzheimer's (incidence), while important, will not directly affect the total burden of care that the community must address. More important is the total number of cases (new and existing) relative to the population. In this example, prevalence becomes the measure of disease frequency that is most relevant to clinicians, health administrators, and policymakers because it informs them of the resources needed to treat the condition at the community or population level in a way that incidence can not.

Perri et al.[4] examined the prevalence of inappropriate medication use within a sample of nursing homes in Georgia identified as high risk for polypharmacy. Medical records were reviewed in 15 nursing homes for evidence of inappropriate medication use, which was defined as any drug within the medical record that met the Beers criteria, a recognized list of potentially inappropriate medications for the elderly.[5] Data were abstracted by chart review for a 1-month period at each institution sometime between March 1 and May 31, 2002. A total of 1,117 patient medical records were reviewed. From this total, 519 patients received at least one inappropriate medication based on the criteria. The 1-month period prevalence was 46.5% (519/1,117).

Relationship Between Incidence and Prevalence

The relationship between incidence and prevalence may be depicted in Figure 2.2. The figure is a bucket that holds water, where the water represents cases. The bucket has an opening at the top for water inflow and two openings at the bottom for water outflow. The water in the bucket at any one time represents all cases, both new and existing, of a disease or condition. This number would be the value within the numerator of a prevalence measure, with the denominator being the number of people in the population at the time cases were recorded. The inflow of water at the top of the bucket represents the new cases that are recorded during some time period. For presentation purposes, those cases are located at the top of the volume of water, although, in reality they are commingled with all cases. The water that has flowed into the bucket over some period of time represents the new cases, and would serve as the numerator in a measure of incidence. The bucket has two openings in which water can flow from the bucket. One opening removes water (cases) from the bucket as the result of disease cure. The second opening removes water (cases) from the bucket as a result of death. If a person had a disease or condition, but had either died or been cured prior to our measurement of the water in the bucket, the person would not be included in the measure of prevalence.

This relationship results in some interesting interpretation of incidence and prevalence values. Recent advances in pharmacotherapy have reduced the number of AIDS deaths and slowed the transition from HIV to AIDS. The Center for Disease Control and Prevention reported a decline of new AIDS cases from 49,999 in 1997 to 41,849 in 1999, and a reduction in AIDS deaths from 22,067 to 16,765 in 1999. More effective treatment has also resulted in an increase in the number of people living with AIDS from 274,624 in 1998 to 322,865 in 2000 (Table 2.2). The consequence of improved prevention and treatment may be a decrease in incidence, but also a commensurate increase in prevalence. Although increased prevalence may appear alarming, increased prevalence of a chronic condition, especially one that has a significant mortality rate, may indicate the success of the intervention employed. Conversely, decreased prevalence might indicate a problem with treatment or care if the decrease is due to an increasing mortality rate (outflow of water that prevents the cases from being included in the prevalence measure). Caution should be exercised and thought given to the interpretation of both incidence and prevalence measures.

Figure 2.2 also implies that incidence and prevalence are related in a way that includes the measurement of time. Prevalence will be affected both by the rate of flow of water into and out of the

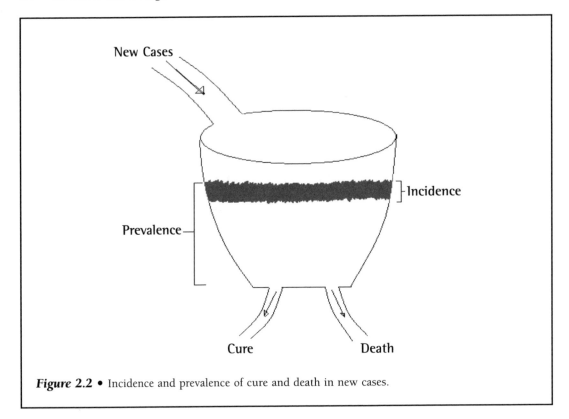

Figure 2.2 • Incidence and prevalence of cure and death in new cases.

Table 2.2
Interpreting Incidence and Prevalence

	1997	1998	1999	2000
AIDS cases	49,999	43,183	41,849	—
AIDS deaths	22,067	18,214	16,765	—
People living with AIDS	—	274,624	299,944	322,865

Source: Centers for Disease Control and Prevention. www.cdc.gov/nchstp/od/news/At-a-Glance.pdf

bucket. Another way of expressing this relationship is that prevalence depends on how long the water stays in the bucket. This concept is termed "duration." In effect, incidence and prevalence are linked in some way to duration. Prevalence is proportional to the incidence rate and the average duration of the disease or condition. Where the inflow and outflow rates are stable (referred to as *steady state,* meaning no dramatic changes in the number of new cases or treatment affecting cure or death rates) and the prevalence of the disease or condition is relatively low, the relationship between incidence and prevalence can be expressed mathematically as:

$$P = I \times D$$

where P = prevalence, I = incidence, and D = duration. This equation allows the assessment of duration of disease, if incidence and prevalence are known. Duration, therefore, can be calculated by dividing prevalence by incidence.

$$D = \frac{P}{I}$$

A hypothetical example demonstrates this relationship. Recently, there have been concerns regarding a strain of virus causing HIV that is resistant to current therapies. If the incidence rate of HIV with this resistant strain is 20 cases/100,000 population/year, and the prevalence of that type of HIV is 7 cases/ 100,000 population, the duration of disease would be calculated as follows:

$$D\ \frac{P}{I} = \frac{7/100,000}{20/100,000/\text{year}} = 0.35\ \text{year}$$

The duration of disease is 0.35 years, or approximately 128 days (0.35 years × 365 days/year). This would indicate that from the date of diagnosis, a person would survive, on average, 128 days. Comparison of disease duration between those with the resistant strain and those with the nonresistant strain would provide insight into the relative virulence of the resistant strain.

Characteristic-Specific Incidence and Prevalence

Up to this point, the discussion of incidence and prevalence has assumed that the reference group is the entire population, i.e., the denominator should include all people in the population at a given time or over a period of time. In fact, measures of disease frequency can be more meaningful if they pertain to specific and relevant segments of the population. For example, one can calculate the incidence of dementia within a population, with the entire population being represented in the denominator. However, because the condition is age-related, with few cases observed before the age of 40, a more meaningful measure may be the incidence of dementia among the subset of the population 40 years of age and older. The same reasoning applies to the measure of prevalence. In either measure, the numerator would include only the cases in which the person was at least 40 years of age. The denominator would include all people who were 40 years of age or older at the time of measurement, and were at risk to develop dementia during the time in question These types of measures of disease frequency are called characteristic-specific incidence or prevalence, where the characteristic can be age, gender, race, disease, or any number of different characteristics. These rates are similar to population rates except that they have been restricted to a particular characteristic of the person or disease of interest. An example is found in Table 2.3. The Health Department of a city of 1,000,000 reports 5,000 cases during the year, for a 1-year incidence of influenza of 500 cases per 100,000 people. However, the rates are much different within different age strata. For brevity, let's segment the population into two age groups, those younger than 50 and those 50 and above, and assume that each stratum contains 500,000 people. Further, assume that the lower age group had 1,000 cases of influenza, while the higher age group had the remaining 4,000 cases. While the overall annual incidence rate is 500 cases/ 100,000 population/year, the age-specific annual incidence rates would be 200 cases/100,000

Table 2.3
Age-Specific Influenza Incidence Rates

	N	Cases	Annual Incidence
Population age groups	1,000,000	5,000	500 per 100,000
0–49	500,000	1,000	200 per 100,000
50+	500,000	4,000	800 per 100,000

population/year and 800 cases/100,000 population/year, respectively. The age-specific incidence rates provide valuable information regarding the susceptibility of different segments of the population. Leary and Saver[6] examined age-specific incidence rates of first silent stroke in the U.S. The authors reported an annual incidence of first silent MRI infarct of 1,600 cases/100,000 population in the 30–39 year age group, and 16,400 cases/100,000 population in the 75–79 year age group. These age-specific rates can assist in the most effective allocation of resources for prevention, education, and treatment.

Mortality

Mortality is an outcome of great interest for several reasons. First, it is a measure of the severity of a clinical condition. Second, it can be useful as a global measure of public health, especially when examining mortality trends. Third, it has great social impact on families and society. Although death should be an easily-identifiable outcome, the aggregation and interpretation of death statistics can be problematic. For a full description of these issues, the reader is referred to Gordis.[7]

Information about mortality can be presented in many ways, and for a variety of purposes. Three methods frequently observed in the literature are described below, each successive one being more specific and providing a different type of information.

Mortality Rates

The most general way to report mortality is to divide the number of deaths during a specified period of time in a population by the number of people in the population during that period.

$$\text{Mortality rate} = \frac{\text{Number of death in a specified time period}}{\text{Number of people in the population during the time period}}$$

Because the size of population is ever-changing, the denominator is some measure of the average population during the time period, e.g., the population mean (beginning plus ending/2), or, population at midpoint in time. If the time period is 1 year, the calculated mortality rate is an annual rate. If the time period is 5 years, the mortality rate is a 5-year mortality rate.

Mortality rates provide a measure of the likelihood of dying during the time period studied. If the mortality rate includes all deaths regardless of cause or reason, the rate is called an all-cause mortality rate. As mentioned above, rates can be restricted to a particular person or disease characteristic, or a combination of characteristics. A clinical researcher might be interested in the annual mortality rate from Reye's Syndrome among children less than 10 years of age. The formula to calculate this age and disease-specific mortality rate is:

$$\text{Mortality rate} = \frac{\text{Number of deaths from Reye's Syndrome among children <10 years of age in 1 year}}{\text{Number of children <10 years of age in population at midyear point}}$$

It is important to remember that the denominator is populated by persons who satisfy the restriction criteria: less than 10 years of age and who had the potential to become cases during the time period.

Mortality rates provide information on the likelihood that a person in the population will die, or will die from a particular disease or condition. These rates are valuable because they make comparisons of mortality rates across different diseases straightforward. For example, mortality rates for many diseases for children less than 10 years of age will have different numerators, representing the number of deaths attributed to each respective disease. The denominators, however, are the same. Because of this, an examination of the number of deaths provides a useful relative comparison of mortality across disease among children.

Case Fatality Rates

Mortality information can also be presented as case fatality rates. Case fatality rates assess the rate at which people who have a particular disease or condition die. The difference between disease-specific mortality rates and case fatality rates are subtle, but substantial. In both rates, the numerator is the number of people who die from a certain disease within the relevant time period. The difference between the two rates lies in the denominator. The denominator of a mortality rate is the number of people in the population at the midpoint of the time studies. These people can be from the entire population, or be restricted to a particular age group, as shown in the example of Reye's Syndrome mortality rate among children less than 10 years of age. The denominator of a case fatality rate is the number of people who have the disease or condition being studied. In effect, the case fatality rate is the rate at which people who have the disease die. As with all rates, the important similarity between mortality and case fatality rates is that every person in the denominator must have the possibility of transitioning to the numerator. Following the example above, the denominator of the mortality rate for Reye's Syndrome must be populated by all children less than 10 years of age who had the possibility of dying from Reye's Syndrome during the relevant time period. The denominator of the case fatality rate for Reye's Syndrome must be populated by all children less than 10 years of age who had Reye's Syndrome and had the possibility of dying from it.

$$\text{Case fatality rate} = \frac{\text{Number of deaths from a specific condition}}{\text{Number of people with the disease or condition}}$$

Generally, most rates will include a specified time period. Case fatality rates, however, typically omit any reference to a specified time period. The main reason is that case fatality rates are used mostly in acute, short-term conditions in which death can be directly attributed to the condition. If death occurs, it will typically be close in time to the initial diagnosis. It makes little sense to calculate and refer to case fatality rates for chronic diseases in which death may be attributed to the disease, but may occur 30 years postdiagnosis.

Proportionate Mortality

Proportionate mortality provides a different way to present mortality information. It is unique in that it does not require a measurement of the size of the population in which deaths occurred. Instead of the denominator being the number of people in the population, it is the total number of deaths in the population over a specified period of time. The numerator is the number of deaths attributed to a particular disease.

$$\text{Proportionate mortality} = \frac{\text{Number of deaths attributed to a disease within a time period}}{\text{Total number of deaths in the population within a time period}}$$

The objective of proportionate mortality measures is to determine the percentage of deaths attributed to a particular disease. An example of such a statement is that 20 percent of all deaths in the U.S. are due to accidents. Proportionate mortality can also be restricted to specific ages, races, geographic regions, etc. For example, by dividing the number of deaths from Sudden Infant Death Syndrome (SIDS) among children 0–1 years of age to all death among children in this age group, one can determine the proportionate mortality of SIDS within this population.

While proportionate mortality provides valuable information, it must be used and interpreted with caution. Unlike other measures, the value of the calculated proportionate mortality is dependent not only on mortality associated with the disease or condition in question, but all other diseases or conditions as well. Using the example above, the calculated value for the proportionate mortality of SIDS is influenced not only by the number of deaths attributed to sudden infant death, but by the number of deaths attributed to all other diseases or conditions that occurred within the 0–1 year age group. The proportionate mortality of SIDS in 2004 might be 10 percent, meaning that 10 percent of all deaths in this age group were due to SIDS. In 2005, the proportionate mortality of SIDS in 2005 might be 2 percent. This dramatic and significant decrease can be misleading, because it may be influenced by external factors that have nothing to do with prevention and educational efforts related to the condition. An increase in deaths attributed to influenza, cancer, etc., could have been the reason for the dramatic decline in sudden infant death proportionate mortality.

Given this limitation, proportionate mortality still provides useful information. It is used frequently to assess the state of health and relative severity of conditions among members of different worker groups (migrant workers) or different patient groups (cancer patients). Proportionate mortality could demonstrate, for example, that accidents account for 40 percent of all deaths among migrant workers, or that lung cancer accounts for 25 percent of all deaths from cancer in the U.S. during a particular time period.

Age-Adjusted Mortality Rates

It is not unusual for clinicians or researchers to compare mortality rates observed at different times. Public health officials might compare mortality rates in different geographic areas to determine the relative health of the population in those areas. Clinicians might compare rates over time within a particular facility to assess the quality of care provided over time. It would appear that the simplest way to do this would be to calculate mortality rates at each time period and compare them directly. Such a comparison, though intuitively appealing, ignores a fundamental requirement for such comparisons to be valid, namely, that the populations must be similar for the comparison to be meaningful and appropriate. If the populations differ significantly on a variable that might affect the rate being calculated, the results could reflect more the influence of the variable that is different in each population and related to the outcome of death than the disease or condition being assessed.

In an ideal world, populations would be similar so that such comparisons could be made. In reality, though, populations are seldom similar, yet there still exists a need to compare them. The solution to this dilemma is to create a method to standardize the mortality rates so that they are comparable. Adjustment of mortality rates relies on an existing or created standard population and an adjustment of characteristic-specific rates. The characteristic can be any variable that is suspected of influencing the mortality rates in the compared populations and unequally distributed across the populations being compared. The characteristic most frequently adjusted in mortality rate comparisons is age because of its strong relationship with mortality. The two hypothetical examples below used to demonstrate both direct and indirect age adjustment will use age-adjusted mortality rates.

Direct Method of Age Adjustment

This method of age adjustment is used to compare mortality rates in populations with different age distributions. In the direct method, the age-specific mortality rates of a study population are applied to the age distribution of a standard population to yield the number of expected deaths in each age group within the standard population. The sum of the expected deaths divided by the total number of people in the standard population results in an age-adjusted mortality rate. In effect, the direct method allows you to determine the number of deaths that would have occurred in the standard population if the age-specific mortality rates of the study population were used.

Mortality rates that do *not* account for age distribution are *crude rates*. The rates are calculated by dividing the total number of deaths by the total population. The 2003 crude mortality rate for South Carolina counties indicated that the counties along the coast had higher crude mortality rates than any other region. One such county, Horry County, had the highest crude mortality rate of all coastal counties, and all counties of South Carolina. Horry County's 2003 crude mortality rate was 12.3 deaths per 1,000 people. South Carolina's 2003 crude mortality rate was 8.2 deaths per 1,000 people. There was great public concern about the quality of health care in a county that would have such an elevated mortality rate.

Table 2.4 presents the data and calculation necessary to construct age-adjusted mortality rates using the direct method. Three variables are necessary: (1) age-specific mortality rates for the study population (Horry County), (2) age distribution of a standard population (South Carolina, 2000), and (3) the expected number of deaths in the standard population in each age category (calculated by multiplying age-specific mortality and age distribution for each age category). The data show that the age-adjusted mortality rate for Horry County was 8.1 per 1,000 people. This is the mortality rate we would expect to observe in the 2000 standard population if the age distribution of Horry County were the same as the age distribution of South Carolina in 2000.

Horry County's crude mortality rate was 12.3, and its age-adjusted mortality rate was 8.1. This discrepancy was due to a higher percentage of older people residing in the county than in the standard

Table 2.4
Horry County Mortality: Direct Method of Age Adjustment

Age Groups	Age-Specific Mortality Rates, Horry County, 2003 (per 1,000)	Age Distribution 2000 SC Population	Expected Deaths
0–4	2.41	310,157	747
5–14	0.16	879,444	141
15–24	1.03	902,687	930
25–34	1.74	741,338	1,290
35–44	3.66	602,985	2,207
45–54	5.31	592,704	3,147
55–64	15.47	413,322	6,394
65–74	31.98	264,697	8,465
75–84	65.58	101,189	6,636
85+	157.23	58,716	9,232
		4,867,239	39,189

Horry County crude mortality rate = 12.3 deaths per 1,000 people (given)
Horry County age-adjusted mortality rate = Expected death/2000 SC population; = 39,189/4,867,239; = 0.0081 = 8.1 deaths per 1,000 people

population of South Carolina; Horry County has a higher crude mortality rate because it has a higher percentage of older people, who, because of their age, have a greater likelihood of dying. This should not be surprising because the coastal areas of South Carolina are attractive places for retirement. Horry County's age-adjusted mortality rate of 8.1 was similar to the overall mortality rate in South Carolina of 8.2 in 2000. If the 2000 South Carolina population were used by all counties as a standard population, direct comparison of age-adjusted mortality rates across counties would be possible. Such a comparison is not appropriate using crude mortality rates. The age-adjusted Horry County mortality rate provides for more appropriate comparison with other counties in South Carolina. Concern should be raised if one of the coastal counties had an age-adjusted mortality rate that remained significantly higher than the mortality rate of the standard population of South Carolina or other counties. This would indicate that the higher mortality rate could not be attributed to a higher percentage of older people in the population.

Indirect Method of Age-Adjustment

This method of age adjustment is frequently used when the number of deaths within each age group in the study population is too small to calculate stable age-specific rates, or the age-specific mortality rates of the study population are unknown. The variables necessary to use the indirect method of age adjustment are the (1) age-specific mortality rates for the standard population population, (2) age distribution of the study population, (3) expected deaths in the study population, and (4) standard mortality ratio, defined as the number of death observed in the study population divided by the number of deaths expected in the study population.

A second hypothetical situation uses the indirect method of age adjustment. Greenville County in South Carolina recently implemented a community-wide program to increase access to health care. The program targeted low income residents who had at least two chronic diseases. One of the goals of the program was to reduce mortality rate within the county.

A simple approach to assessing the effectiveness of the program would be to compare the crude mortality rates of Greenville County in 2000 with the rates in 2005. However, because the county has experienced significant growth since 2000, it was considered appropriate to calculate and compare age-adjusted mortality rates, because Greenville County's age distribution may have changed in the intervening period. The population of Greenville County in 2000 serves as the standard population, and the population in 2005 serves as the study population. The indirect method of age-adjustment was used because, at the time to evaluate the program, the 2005 age-specific mortality rates in Greenville County were not available.

Table 2.5 presents the necessary data for the calculation of age-specific mortality rates using the indirect method. The age-specific mortality rates of the standard population (Greenville, 2000) are applied to the age distribution of the study population (Greenville, 2005). The multiplication yields the number of deaths expected in the study population in each age group. The sum of the age-specific expected deaths gives the number of deaths expected in Greenville County in 2005 if the age-specific mortality rates of Greenville County in 2000 are applied. The number of observed deaths (actual deaths recorded) is divided by the expected deaths to yield the Standardized Mortality Ratio. There were 2,237 expected deaths in Greenville County in 2005 if the age-specific mortality rates of 2000 were applied to the 2005 population. Health department records indicate that there were 2,019 actual deaths among residents of the county. The Standard Mortality Ratio is 0.90 (2,019/2,237). The number of deaths in Greenville County in 2005 were 90 percent of what was expected, adjusted for the effects

Table 2.5
Horry County Mortality: Indirect Method of Age-Adjustment

Age Groups	Age-Specific Mortality Rates, SC, 2000 (Per 1,000)	Age Distribution of Greenville County, 2005	Expected Deaths
0–4	1.94	27,329	53
5–14	0.13	51,081	7
15–24	1.02	50,367	51
25–34	1.63	47,649	78
35–44	2.37	52,323	124
45–54	4.69	38,187	179
55–64	15.44	29,005	448
65–74	27.32	20,811	569
75–84	70.04	18,475	129
85+	138.56	4,320	599
		339,547	2,237

Deaths in Greenville County in 2005 = 2,019 (given)
Standard Mortality Ratio = 2,019/2,237 = 0.90

of age. These results would be viewed as suggestive evidence that the program may have been successful in reducing mortality.

Summary

This chapter established the fundamental role of counting in our attempt to understand the world about us. In health care, counting events, whether they be diseases, hospitalizations, or adverse drug reactions, and reporting them within a clear and understandable context, is critical to gaining this understanding. In the most general sense, we create rates and proportions to avoid the problems with numerator analysis. In epidemiology and outcomes research, the measure of disease or outcome frequency, using either rates or proportions, is captured in the assessment of incidence and prevalence. Incidence is the number of new cases or events in a population over a specified period of time divided by the population at risk, while prevalence is the number of existing cases or events in a population at a particular point or period of time, divided by the population at risk. Incidence may be reported as cumulative incidence or incidence density. Prevalence may be reported as point prevalence or period prevalence. In a steady state, incidence and prevalence are related to each other through a measure of the duration of disease. Incidence and prevalence can be reported for the population of interest or for particular subsets of the population, e.g., the population stratified by age, gender, race, income, etc.

Mortality is an outcome used in epidemiology and outcomes research that warrants particular attention. It is reported in a variety of ways, including overall mortality rate, case fatality rate, and proportionate mortality. Most measures of mortality include some adjustment for potential confounding factors. Because death is so strongly related to age, age-specific rates are frequently reported. This adjustment allows comparison of rates across different groups.

The counting of events, and the calculation of incidence and prevalence, is relevant to topics covered throughout this book. The count of events or outcomes in groups exposed to factors of interest, e.g., drugs, interventions, etc., can be compared to the count of events or outcomes in groups not exposed to these factors of interest. This comparison is the basis of the calculation of relative risks and odds ratios covered in the chapter on research design. The calculated risk of events in the population is used in decision tree analysis, again covered in a subsequent chapter.

Happy counting!

References

1. Wong TY, Rosamond W, Chang PP, Couper DJ, Sharrett AR, Hubbard LD, Folsom AR, Klein R. Retinopathy and risk of congestive heart failure. *JAMA.* 2005;292(1):63–69.
2. Lacoste-Roussillon C, Pouyanne P, Haramburu F, Miremont G, Begaud B. Incidence of serious adverse reactions in general practice: A prospective study. *Clin Pharm Ther.* 2001;69:458–462.
3. Van Roon EN, Jansen TLThA, Mourad L, Houtman PM, Bruyn GAW, Griep EN, Wilffert B, Tobi H, Brouwers JRBJ. Leflunomide in active rheumatoid arthritis: a prospective study in daily practice. *Br J Clin Pharm.* 2004;57(6):790–797.
4. Perri III M, Menon AM, Deshpande AP, Shinde SB, Jiang R, Cooper JW, Cook CL, Griffin SC, Lorys RA. Adverse outcomes associated with inappropriate drug use in nursing homes. *Ann Pharmacother.* 2005;39:405–411.
5. Beers MH. Explicit criteria for determining potentially inappropriate medication use by the elderly: an update. *Archiv Intern Med.* 1997;157:1531–1536.
6. Leary MC, Saver JL. Annual incidence of first silent stroke in the U.S.: a preliminary estimate. *Cerebrovasc Dis.* 2003;16(3):280–285.
7. Gordis L. *Epidemiology.* 2nd ed. Philadelphia: W.B. Saunders Company; 2000.

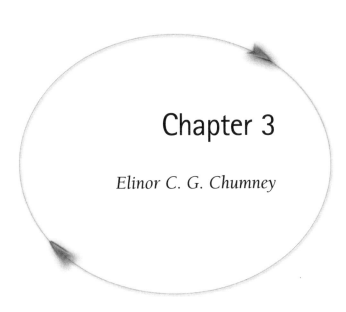

Chapter 3

Elinor C. G. Chumney

Ecologic Analysis

The Japanese eat very little fat and suffer fewer heart attacks than the British or the Americans. But then the French eat a lot of fat and also suffer fewer heart attacks than we do. The Japanese drink very little red wine and suffer fewer heart attacks than the British or the Americans. But then the Italians drink excessive amounts of red wine and they, too, suffer fewer heart attacks than we do. What are we to conclude from all of this? In short, you can eat and drink what you like. Speaking English is apparently what kills you.

(*Readers' Digest,* September 2003)

As we will learn in later chapters of this section, case-control, cohort, and randomized clinical trials all focus on comparisons of individuals. Information for these analyses is often gathered through individual interviews or medical records and is specific for each person included in the sample. These individual-level approaches are relatively labor-intensive and expensive, but they are routinely conducted because they allow researchers to predict individual risk or odds.

By comparison, ecologic or aggregate analyses focus on comparisons of groups. Typically the groups are derived from geographically defined areas, such as nations, states, or counties, and the analyses combine existing datasets on these large populations.

Ecologic analyses look at aggregated data such as percentages, rates, and means. These data may be classified into three main types[1]:

1. Aggregate measures or summaries of observations derived from individuals in a group (e.g., national literacy rates, state cancer rates, county employment rates, or class average SAT scores)
2. Environmental measures or characteristics of the place in which the individuals in the group live or work (e.g., average environmental toxin levels or mean hours of sunlight)
3. Global measures (e.g., the existence of a specific law, the type of health care system, and population density)

Ecologic analyses then use these data to predict group rates of outcomes such as disease. The most common method of analysis for ecologic data is ordinary least squares (OLS) or linear regression, which we will cover in greater detail in Chapter 9.[1] The dependent variable (Y) is then the group-specific disease rate or prevalence, and the independent variables (Xs) are group-specific exposure prevalences.

Example

Consider a recent analysis by Gross and colleagues that examined the relationship between the increased consumption of refined carbohydrates and the prevalence of type 2 diabetes in the United States between 1933 and 1997.[2] They obtained estimates of the prevalence of diabetes in the U.S. from the National Health Interview Surveys maintained by the Centers for Disease Control and Prevention's Diabetes Surveillance System.[3] The nutrient content of the U.S. food supply was obtained from the National Nutrient Data Bank, which is maintained by the Center for Nutrition Policy and Promotion and the Economic Research Service of the U.S. Department of Agriculture.[4]

In their linear regression model, Gross and colleagues found a strong and statistically significant association between an increasing trend in the prevalence of type 2 diabetes and both an increased consumption of refined carbohydrates in the form of corn syrup (β = 0.0132, p = 0.038) and a decreased consumption of dietary fiber (β = −13.86, p < 0.01) in the U.S. during the 20th century (see Table 3.1 and Figure 3.1). For further information on interpreting the results of linear regression analyses, please refer to Chapter 9.

Advantages of Ecologic Analyses

Ecologic analyses have several practical advantages that make them especially appealing for certain types of research and have led to their widespread use in epidemiology:

Table 3.1
Linear Regression Model Examining the Associations Between Trends in Nutrients and the Prevalence of Type 2 Diabetes in the U.S. Between 1933 and 1997

Nutrient contribution	β Coefficient	P
Dietary fiber (% of energy)	−13.86	0.0083
Corn syrup (% of energy)	0.0132	0.038
Protein (% of energy)	−3.58	0.084
Fat (% of energy)	0.00196	0.79
Total energy (kcal)	0.00011	0.28

A positive β coefficient indicates an increased risk of type 2 diabetes, whereas a negative coefficient indicates a decreased risk of type 2 diabetes.

Source: Reproduced with permission by the American Journal of Clinical Nutrition. *Am J Clin Nutr.* © American Society for Clinical Nutrition.

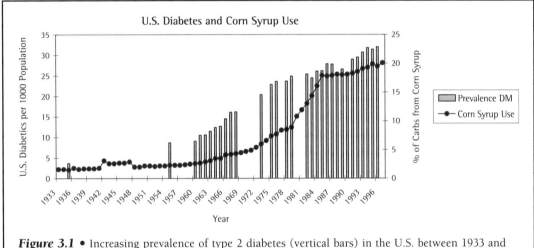

Figure 3.1 • Increasing prevalence of type 2 diabetes (vertical bars) in the U.S. between 1933 and 1997 with increasing per capita percentage of carbohydrate intake from corn syrup.

Source: Reproduced with permission by the American Journal of Clinical Nutrition. *Am J Clin Nutr.* © American Society for Clinical Nutrition.

1. *They are quick, convenient, and inexpensive.* Because they are often based on existing (i.e., secondary) data that is publicly available, such as the two datasets employed by Gross and colleagues[2] in our first example, ecologic analyses are generally less expensive and take less time than individual-level analyses.

2. *They are ideally suited to generate hypotheses.* Because they are so quick and inexpensive, they are often used to explore potential relationships between diseases and exposures and provide theoretical support for individual-level studies of the same issue.

3. *They avoid some of the measurement limitations of individual-level studies.* There are many variables that are difficult to accurately measure at an individual level and are far easier to get on an aggregated level. For example, obtaining accurate annual carbohydrate consumption figures for individuals in a study population would be an extraordinarily complex, expensive, and time-consuming undertaking. By contrast, Gross and colleagues were able to substitute for this measure with a readily available estimate of per capita carbohydrate consumption based on national food disappearance data.[2]

In fact, many individual level studies are now routinely incorporating some ecologic or group-level measurements in their analyses.[5] This is especially true in environmental epidemiology, where researchers are unable to accurately measure relevant exposures or doses at the individual level for large numbers of subjects—at least not with available time and resources. Thus, an ecologic measurement may be the only practical way to approximate a measure of the exposure of interest.[1,6] We will discuss multi-level analyses later in this chapter.

4. *They are ideally suited to evaluate the population effect of public policies, programs, and legislation.* Ecologic analyses are especially well-suited for evaluating issues from a public health perspective, such as policy analyses evaluating the effectiveness of a community intervention. Because legislation is applied to an entire population, it is actually more informative to analyze the effect on the group. For example, researchers could use an ecologic analysis to assess the effect of gun safety laws on state murder rates or the effect of flu vaccine clinics on employee workdays missed.

Limitations of Ecologic Analyses

It is especially important to keep in mind the limitations of an ecologic analysis.

1. *Avoid the ecologic fallacy.* Mistakenly concluding that because an association exists between exposure and disease at the group level it also exists at the individual level is known as the "ecologic fallacy." It is the failure of ecologic effect estimates to reflect biologic effects at the individual level. Because the data in ecologic studies are measurements aggregated over individuals, the associations between exposure and disease at the group level do not necessarily reflect individual-level associations. The basic problem is heterogeneity within groups.

   Suppose a researcher finds that national breast cancer mortality rates tend to be higher in countries with high-fat diets using ecologic data. If, based on this analysis alone, he or she were then to infer that individuals with high-fat diets are more likely to have breast cancer, he or she would be committing an ecologic fallacy. Because only group-level variables were used in the analysis, the researcher would have no way of knowing whether the breast cancer he or she observed occurring in nations with high fat consumption was actually occurring among women who are consuming a lot of fat. The citation at the beginning of this chapter serves as another more humorous illustration of this very common problem with ecologic analyses.

2. *Restricted to available data.* Another chief limitation of ecologic analyses is that they are restricted to available data. For example, the analysis of type 2 diabetes by Gross and colleagues used data from the National Nutrition Databank.[2] These nutrient data are based on annual food disappearance in the United States over the last century and are the foundation of essentially all public and private work in the field of human nutrition.[2] However, food disappearance data at the population level are only an indirect measure of individual consumption.

   As in the previous section, suppose that a researcher finds that national breast cancer mortality rates tend to be higher in countries with high-fat diets using ecologic data. It would be important to note that the researcher used readily available mortality data, instead of the preferred incidence data. Because treatment and access can vary dramatically across countries, it is possible that disease rates were actually the same between the countries but that different levels of health care led to higher detection or death rates in some countries.

3. *Overall correlations can mask important differences in subgroups.* As in the previous sections, suppose that the same researcher noted a number of important outliers in his analysis of national breast

cancer mortality rates and dietary fat. In particular, he found that Mediterranean countries tended towards a relatively high per capita fat consumption, yet their breast cancer mortality rates were much lower than would be expected based on the cross-national data. The fact that olive oil is the predominate source of fat in these countries has helped to fuel the notion that the type as well as the amount of dietary fat typical of a nation's diet may be an important determinant of future public health.

Multi-Level Analyses

After discovering the ecologic fallacy, early epidemiologists and public health researchers at first tended to shy away from ecologic analyses and data altogether. Later they used ecologic analyses to generate hypotheses and tended to trust the results only when they were supported by individual-level analyses, such as a case-control study.

Today, there is a growing appreciation for the merits of ecologic analyses, especially given the increased awareness in the research community that not all disease determinants can be conceptualized as individual-level attributes.[5] Ecologic or group-level variables may be used as proxies for unavailable individual-level data.

Increasingly, they are also being used because of the potential health effects of group-level constructs, such as income inequality, neighborhood characteristics, environmental factors, and the presence of certain public health policies.[5] Many individual-level analyses now routinely incorporate some ecologic measurements. These so-called multi-level analyses extend beyond the study of individual epidemiological factors by simultaneously incorporating different levels of variables (i.e., individual, workplace, neighborhood, community, or region) that might influence an individual's state of health.[7] They can then assess whether individual health is shaped by group-level variables such as household (e.g., family income) or population characteristics (e.g., population density or the proportion of people living in poverty).[7]

Conclusion

Ecologic analyses have several practical advantages that make them especially appealing for certain types of research. These include the fact that (1) individual-level data is often missing or unreliable, (2) they are perfectly suited for the public health perspective, examining the population effect of legislation or other interventions, and (3) they are quick, convenient, and inexpensive, using readily available data. But ecologic analyses must be interpreted cautiously at the individual/biological level to avoid the "ecologic fallacy."

References

1. Morgenstern H. Ecologic studies. In: Rothman KJ, Greenland S, eds. *Modern Epidemiology.* 2nd ed. Philadelphia: Lippincott; 1998:459–80.
2. Gross LS, Li Li, Ford ES, et al. Increased consumption of refined carbohydrates and the epidemic of type 2 diabetes in the United States: an ecologic assessment. *Am J Clin Nutr.* 2004;79(5):774–79.
3. Centers for Disease Control and Prevention, National Center for Health Statistics, Division of Health Interview Statistics. Census of the population and population estimates. Hyattsville, MD: Centers for Disease Control and Prevention, 1997.
4. U.S. Department of Agriculture, Center for Nutrition Policy and Promotion. Nutrient content of the U.S. food supply. Version current 29 May 2003 (accessed 3 February 2004).

5. Roux AVD. The study of group-level factors in epidemiology: rethinking variables, study designs, and analytical approaches. *Epidemiol Rev.* 2004;26:104–11.

6. Morgenstern H. Uses of ecological analysis in epidemiologic research. *Am J Public Healh.* 1982;72(12):1336–44.

7. Krieger N. A glossary for social epidemiology. *J Epidemiol Community Health.* 2001;55(10):693–700.

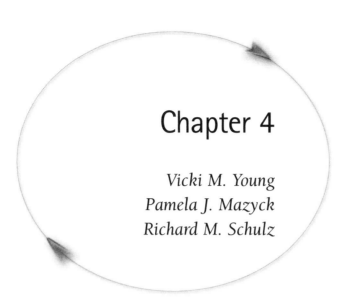

Chapter 4

Vicki M. Young
Pamela J. Mazyck
Richard M. Schulz

Epidemiologic Study Designs

Introduction

Clinicians have a professional obligation to attend to the health care needs of their patients. They use information from a variety of sources to make informed decisions regarding that care. For clinicians and nonclinicians alike, personal experience serves as a powerful teacher. The nurse who has successfully used specific verbal and nonverbal techniques to reach a noncommunicative patient will incorporate these techniques into his or her professional practice. The pharmacist who has observed drug interactions with a particular combination of medicines will communicate that concern and provide a warning to others. Clinicians also learn from experts or opinion leaders. Attending professional conferences or observing the practice patterns of recognized leaders in one's area provides the benefit of hearing the views and observing the decisions of these opinion leaders.

A third way health professionals develop excellence in the care of their patients is by reading and assimilating the professional literature relevant to their practices. The development of practice guidelines and evidence-based medicine is an organizational and behavioral response to the information presented in the literature. However, health professionals are assaulted daily by an avalanche of information. Shenk[1] chronicles this situation in the general population in his book, *Data Smog*. Within the health professions, Arndt[2] and Davidoff et al.[3] describe the situation in which health professionals are overwhelmed with information, much of it irrelevant or of little value. The challenge, then, for health professionals is to become most efficient in their ability to distinguish between high and low impact studies for their professional practice. The ability of health professionals to reduce the noise-to-message ratio directly impacts the time and quality of care they can give to their patients.

Knowledge of study design is a quick and effective way to assess the confidence one should have in the results of a published study and its influence on practice behavior. While all study designs have some inherent value, they also have varying degrees of weakness. This chapter will describe various study designs employed frequently in clinical and epidemiologic studies, with a primary focus on case-control and cohort study designs.

Study designs can broadly be characterized as observational or experimental. Observational studies are those in which the investigator observes but does not intervene. Experimental studies are characterized by an investigator intervening in some way, and then observing the results of the intervention. An example of an experimental study familiar to most clinicians is the randomized control trial in which subjects are randomized to either an experimental or control group, receive different exposures (e.g., Drug A or Drug B), and then are compared on some measure (e.g., blood pressure). The randomized control design (discussed in greater detail in Chapter 5) is considered the gold standard of designs because it reduces or eliminates many threats to the validity of the study results. For this and other reasons, we typically have greater confidence in experimental studies. However, greater confidence in the results from a particular design comes at a price. Experimental studies will be more costly in terms of time and money than observational studies. Also, ethical considerations may preclude the use of an experimental design, especially if it involves the use of life-saving interventions. For these reasons, observational studies are also important, useful, and needed. Another price exchange or trade-off between experimental and observational studies occurs as it relates to internal and external validity. Although observational studies compared to experimental studies are considered lacking in the ability to prove internal validity or causality, they may be much stronger when considering external validity or generalizability. This trade-off between internal and external validity can be viewed also as a trade-off between efficacy and effectiveness. Experimental designs, in testing causality, test the internal validity between intervention (exposure) and outcome under controlled conditions. In other words, they test efficacy. Observational studies, which tend to possess external validity, test the ability of an intervention to produce an outcome under natural conditions. This approach examines the effectiveness of an intervention. Studies test either efficacy or effectiveness; observational studies tend to test effectiveness.

Experimental studies are examined in more detail in another chapter in this book. Observational studies are the focus of this chapter, and will be discussed below. Understanding observational and experimental studies and their attendant strengths and limitations will allow clinicians and students alike to better interpret the results of studies using these designs.

Several different types of designs fall under the broad heading of observational studies. They are presented below in order of increasing time and cost to complete, increasing control of threats to validity, and accordingly, increasing confidence in the results.

Case Report and Case Series

A clinician who observes and reports some clinical finding regarding a patient has conducted an observational study called a *case report*. A case series differs from a case report in that it reports the findings regarding several patients. Typically, case reports or case series describe the finding with respect to person, place, time, and other relevant variables. For example, a clinician may describe a patient whose blood pressure rose subsequent to the use of a particular drug. The clinician presents demographic and clinical information about the patient, as well as the time sequence of events. This simple design serves the purpose of introducing an audience to potentially new information about a possible association between the drug and clinical outcome. The author (and reader) should not infer any causal relationship between drug and blood pressure, primarily because the design does not allow for hypothesis testing. This study design does not include a comparison group, nor does it include a randomization of subjects. Therefore, the rise in blood pressure could have a variety of plausible alternative explanations. Although the weakest of the observational study designs, many clinical journals routinely report results of studies using these designs in sections titled "Case Reports." These designs serve the purpose of increasing the readers' awareness of a possible association, thereby potentially motivating others to test the proposed relationship using a stronger design.

Ecologic Studies

Ecologic studies use populations, or naturally occurring groups of people, as the unit of analysis instead of individuals. An example of an ecologic analysis is an examination of the relationship between strokes per 100,000 and use of oral contraceptive per 100,000 in different cities in the United States. A researcher might report a strong positive, linear relationship between the two. But because the unit of analysis is cities instead of individuals, there is no assurance that the people who suffered a stroke were themselves taking oral contraceptives. The erroneous conclusion that can be drawn from studies with this design is termed the "ecologic fallacy." This problem notwithstanding, ecologic studies provide useful information. The strong relationship described above is suggestive enough to warrant further examination. Again, lower level observational studies serve the purpose of sensitizing the clinical community to the possibility of a relationship between two variables of clinical importance. Ecologic analyses were described in more detail in Chapter 3.

Cross-Sectional Studies

Cross-sectional studies provide useful information about the prevalence of a condition or disease at a particular point in time. Data can be collected in a variety of ways, including surveys, chart reviews, and large database analyses. A critical shortcoming of all methods of data collection in cross-sectional studies is that they do not establish a temporal sequence of variables examined. For example, a cross-sectional study can provide valuable information about the prevalence of antidepressant use in a population. Likewise, it can provide prevalence data regarding suicide ideation in a community. However, because temporal sequence cannot be established within the context of a cross-sectional design, the researcher and reader cannot infer that suicide ideation is the result of antidepressant use. Cross-sectional studies cannot answer the question of whether antidepressants precede or follow suicide ideation, because both are assessed simultaneously. As with other observational studies already described, cross-sectional studies provide valuable information that should lead the clinician and reader to suspect that a relationship might exist.

Case–Control Studies

Case-control studies, along with cohort studies, are observational studies that include the significant design improvement of a control group. The presence of a control group addresses several possible threats to internal validity. For example, no longer can a clinical outcome be attributed to the aging of the study population as a plausible alternative explanation. Such changes would have occurred in the control group as well. Clinical outcomes should not be attributed to events external to the study if those events affected both groups similarly. It is important to note that the presence of the control group does not automatically eliminate potential confounding events from occurring. Rather, the events *may* affect both groups in a similar fashion, thus negating their effect. If the event affects the two groups differently, much of the value of the control group is lost, and the event may confound the result, i.e., results may be due more to the confounder than to the exposure of interest. Generally, however, the introduction of a control group yields improved internal validity, and allows the reader to have increased confidence in the reported results.

Case-control studies are a type of observational epidemiologic investigation in which subjects are selected on the basis of an outcome or disease of interest. Subjects who have the disease or outcome are called cases. Subjects who do not have the disease or outcome are called controls. Cases can be incident (newly diagnosed) or prevalent (current but previously diagnosed). Cases and controls are then compared with respect to an exposure of interest. A source of confusion concerning case-control studies is that the selection of subjects begins with case or control status (i.e., whether or not the subject has the disease). The researcher then looks backwards in time to assess exposure. The relevant question in case-control studies is whether subjects with the disease or outcome differ from those without the disease or outcome with respect to their exposure (to a drug, surgical technique, diet, method of counseling, etc.).

Selecting Cases

Case-control (as well as cohort) studies require that cases are identified and recorded as precisely as possible. Such ascertainment typically begins with a definition that is logistically linked to the study methodology. For example, a case-control study in which depression is the outcome of interest may use an administrative claims database to identify cases of depression. In this study, all people within the database who have an ICD-9 of 296.2 might be included in the study. This ICD-9 is given to people with major depressive disorders; it excludes other types of depression frequently linked with other diagnoses (for example, 296.5 is bipolar affective disorder, depressed). Alternately, cases of depression may be identified by a particular score on a depression scale, such as the Hamilton or Zung Rating Scales for depression. Within either design or operational definition, people within the control group would be those who failed to satisfy the requirement to be considered a case, i.e., they would not have the requisite ICD-9 or they would not have reached a threshold score for depression.

Exposure Measurement

Precise assessment of the exposure of subjects to the variable of interest is a critical component in case-control and cohort studies. As with the ascertainment of cases, exposure measurement can have a variety of sources. Examples include pharmacy records (to determine drug exposure), diet surveys and diaries (to determine nutritional exposure), and school records (to determine whether subjects were immunized). To avoid bias, the method to obtain exposure information should be similar for all subjects regardless of their being cases or controls. In addition, knowledge of a subject's case status typically is not known by the person collecting or recording information about the subject's exposure.

Selecting Controls

The selection of controls in a case control study can be both conceptually and practically challenging. One misconception about control groups is that they should be mirror images of the case group except for the presence of disease. Another fallacy is that they should represent the population of subjects who do not have the outcome or disease. Rather, the control group should be composed of subjects who are comparable to the source population for cases, and would have been identified as cases if they had developed the disease. Controls must be selected to represent not the entire nondiseased population but the population of individuals who would have been identified and included as cases had they also developed the disease.

A case control study examining the relationship between a new pain medication and the development of ulcers subsequent to surgery may identify cases from the orthopedic service of a hospital. Controls might be selected from the group of people within the hospital who have had surgery. The critical aspect of selecting controls is not that the general surgery patients are the same as the orthopedic patients, or that they represent all people who have had surgeries. The control group, however, must come from the same source population (admitted to the hospital) so that they would have been identified as a case (developed ulcer after surgery) if, in fact, an ulcer developed.

There are several possible sources commonly used, including hospital controls, general population controls, and special control series such as friends, neighbors, or relatives of cases. Each offers particular advantages and disadvantages that must be considered for any particular study in view of the nature of the cases, their source, and the type of information to be obtained. For example, one advantage of using hospitalized patients is that they can be easily identified. The major disadvantage is that these patients are usually very ill. In addition, general population controls can be obtained via random-digit dialing, population registers or voting lists/poll information. Identifying controls from this population presents a disadvantage in that this is a costly method and very time consuming. Finally, special group controls which consist of friends, relatives, etc., tend to be willing participants due to their special interest in the selected case. A more detailed discussion of the advantages and disadvantages of the different sources of control groups can be found in Hennekens and Buring.[4]

Selecting the Number of Control Groups and Subjects

The reader of studies using case-control designs must remember that the control group is created by the investigator. As such, it is the result of decisions the investigator makes. Two of these decisions are the number of control groups and the number of subjects within groups. Typically, the investigator creates one group of controls to be compared to the group of cases. There are situations in which more than one control group is advisable. Generally, an investigator would select more than one control group if there was concern that the first control group might not be entirely appropriate. In the above example, the selection of hospital-wide surgery patients for the control group may be less than appropriate if the group included patients from a gastroenterology service, where patients may have been admitted because of ulcers, or were more prone to developing ulcers. In this situation, the one hospital-wide control group might be less desirable than several groups, each from different services within the hospital (excluding gastroenterology). Consistency in the strength of association across the different control groups would provide evidence that the investigator's decision regarding multiple control groups did not introduce bias.

The number of subjects in the control group is dependent on the availability of subjects for inclusion in the groups, as well as the time and cost associated with identifying them and collecting information about them. Where cases and controls are plentiful and the cost of obtaining information about cases and controls is similar, a ratio of 1:1 is desirable. However, if the number of cases is small and the time and money cost of obtaining information on additional controls is not excessive, additional subjects in the control group is desirable. Increasing the number of subjects in the control group will give the study additional power by reducing estimate variability. Beyond a 4:1 control to case ratio, the increased power resulting from expanding the number of subjects in the control group is negligible.[4]

Measurement of Association

Measures of association are point estimates of the relationship between exposure and outcome. The confidence placed in the point estimate is represented by the confidence interval, which establishes low and high bounds within which the true point estimate lies. All measures of association have confidence intervals associated with them. Confidence intervals are discussed in more detail in the section on cohort studies.

In case-control studies, the association between a disease and an exposure is assessed by calculating an odds ratio. The odds of exposure among cases is compared to the odds of exposure among controls. Dividing the respective odds yields an odds ratio. An odds ratio of 1.0 indicates that the odds of exposure among cases is equal to the odds of exposure among controls. A value greater than 1.0 indicates that the odds of exposure among cases is greater than the odds of exposure among controls. A value less than 1.0 indicates that the odds of exposure among cases is less than the odds of exposure among controls.

In their simplest form, case-control studies can be represented by 2 × 2 tables depicting two levels of disease (yes or no) and two levels of exposure (yes or no). In Table 4.1, "a" represents subjects who had the disease or outcome of interest and who had the exposure; "c" represents subjects who had the disease but were not exposed. The odds of exposure among cases, therefore is represented by the ratio a/c. The same explanation applies to subjects represented by "b" and "d" in the table. The odds ratio, therefore, is the ratio of two odds, a/c divided by b/d.

$$\text{Odds ratio} = a/c \ / \ b/d$$

$$ad \ / \ bc \qquad \text{(equivalent but simpler form of ratio above)}$$

Case-control designs typically involve more than one variable that might affect outcome status. Frequently, these variables are not the main variable of interest, but they are included because they might influence the association between the exposure variable of interest and the outcome variable. If these variables are related to the outcome and are present to different degrees in the two exposure groups, then the variables may be confounders in that they can confound the relationship between the

Table 4.1
2 × 2 Cross-Tabulation of Exposure and Disease in a Case-Control Study

Exposure	Disease	No Disease
Present	a	b
Absent	c	d

exposure and outcome. Investigators can choose from several strategies to control for confounding, including stratification, restriction, and multivariate analysis. A full description of the other methods is beyond the scope of this chapter on designs, and the reader is referred to Hennekens and Buring,[4] Gordis,[5] or Rothman.[6] Multivariate analysis will also be discussed in more detail in Chapters 8, 9, and 10.

Case-Control Study Example

A pharmaceutical company has accumulated evidence from case reports and case series suggesting that its drug for hypertension is protective against developing glaucoma. A case-control study was conducted in which community-based cases of glaucoma were identified. An appropriate control group of subjects without glaucoma was created. The distribution of cases and controls with and without exposure to the hypertension drug is reported in the table below:

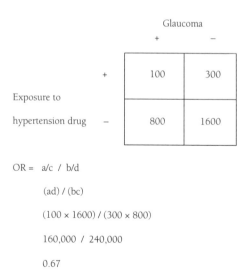

Glaucoma

	+	−
Exposure to hypertension drug +	100	300
−	800	1600

$$OR = a/c \ / \ b/d$$

$$(ad) / (bc)$$

$$(100 \times 1600) / (300 \times 800)$$

$$160,000 \ / \ 240,000$$

$$0.67$$

This case-control study provides additional evidence that supports the hypothesis developed from the case reports and case series, namely, that exposure to the hypertension drug is protective against the development of glaucoma. In this study, people who had glaucoma (the cases) were two-thirds as likely to have been exposed to the hypertension drug as people who did not have glaucoma (the controls).

Case-control studies do not allow for the direct assessment of risk because the population at risk is never known. The control groups are created, and can range from large to small in size. Odds ratios are an approximation of relative risk, especially when the disease is rare. The measure of association in case-control studies is calculated as an odds ratio, but might be reported as a relative risk. The reader should be aware that odds ratios reported in this manner are only an approximation of risk, one necessitated by the case-control design. This relationship can be verified mathematically using the symbols within the 2 × 2 table in Table 4.1. If the disease is rare, then "a" and "c" become very small in value. The calculation of relative risk (a/a+b)/(c/c+d) reduces to (a/b)/(c/d). The values of "b" and "d" dominate the denominator. Relative risk, therefore is (a/b)/(c/d) which can be transformed to ad/bc, the formula listed above for odds ratio.

Strengths and Limitations

Case-control studies have several important strengths and limitations. They are relatively quick and inexpensive when compared to experimental studies. They are appropriate for the evaluation of diseases with long latency periods and for diseases or outcomes that are rare or infrequently observed. Both of these strengths are derived from the fact that case-control studies do not require the investigator to follow subjects over time to determine if the disease or outcome develops. Case-control designs allow the investigator to begin at a point in time when the disease or outcome has already been expressed. However, this aspect of case-control designs also is responsible for their limitation, as well. Case-control designs are prone to bias, especially if subjects are contributing information about exposures through recall. Subjects who have a disease or condition may be more motivated to recall exposures in the past than subjects who do not have the disease. This differential recall is the source of any potential bias. Case-control designs are also inefficient for the study of the relationship between a disease and especially rare exposures. Also, because the investigator categorizes subjects based on the presence or absence of disease, the size of the population at risk is never known. This limitation precludes the direct calculation of incidence rates. The odds ratio serves as an approximation of relative risk.

Cohort Studies

A cohort or follow-up study is an observational design in which a group or groups of individuals are defined on the basis of the presence or absence of exposure to a suspected risk factor for a disease; they are then followed over a period of time to assess the occurrence of the disease.[4] The objective of a cohort study is usually to investigate whether the incidence of a disease event is related to a suspected exposure.[7] Therefore, a cohort study is an observational study where a group of disease-free individuals is identified, exposure to a certain factor determined, and then the individuals in the groups are followed for a specific timeframe to assess the occurrence of the disease or outcome.

When viewed as an analytical process as explored by Szklo and Nieto,[7] the steps involved in the design and conduct of cohort studies are as follows: (1) define the cohort; (2) select or classify the participants based on exposure status; (3) follow participants for a period of time; (4) determine the incidence of disease in the different exposure groups; (5) compare the incidences across exposure groups. This basic analytical approach is depicted schematically in Figure 4.1, where participants (exposed and unexposed) remain in a nondiseased state over time or transition to a diseased state.

Study Population

Study participants can be selected in several ways, which can lead to diverse study populations (7). Participants can be selected from either (1) a defined population or population sample or (2) exposed

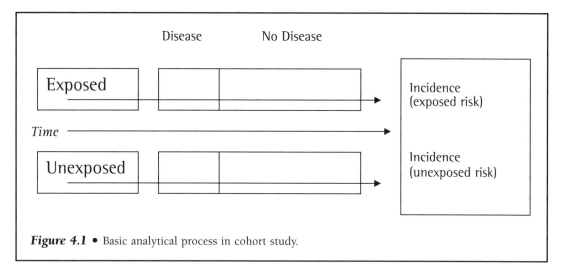

Figure 4.1 • Basic analytical process in cohort study.

Source: Adapted from Szklo M, Nieto FJ. *Epidemiology Beyond the Basics*. Sudbury, MA: Jones and Bartlett Publishers, Inc.; 2000:27.

and unexposed individuals who are then included in the study. Cohorts can also be formed based on logistic advantages. The choice of the appropriate population depends on a variety of factors including, but not restricted to, the frequency of the exposures under study, the need to obtain complete and accurate information on all study participants, and the nature of the problem being examined. If the exposure occurs frequently, then defining the population on the basis of factors not related to exposure first and then ascertaining exposure status is appropriate. Selecting specific study populations (e.g., nurses, veterans, students, employed individuals) based on logistic considerations may facilitate the collection of a higher rate of more accurate exposure and outcome information. One advantage of identifying the exposed and unexposed individuals first is the ability to collect exposure and outcome information on a sufficient number of subjects in a timely manner.

Types of Cohort Studies

Cohort studies are generally categorized as prospective or retrospective. This categorization is based on the point in the analytical process that the study begins. Figure 4.2 illustrates the difference in the categories.

When the cohort is defined before the study starts and then is followed into the future, the cohort study is referred to as prospective. The opportunity for exposure may or may not have occurred at this time, but the outcome definitely has not occurred. This type of prospective cohort study has also been referred to as concurrent.[7] A major advantage of prospective studies is that the methods of ascertaining exposure and outcome status as well as follow-up are planned and implemented for the purpose of the specific study being conducted. The ability to use interviews, questionnaires, examinations, and tests to address the specific research questions posed in the study is also a major advantage but faces the potential of bias based on interviewer objectivity. Blinding the examiner or interviewer to the study purpose can diminish this form of bias. Disadvantages of prospective studies involve the amount of time and resources (funding) needed to conduct the study. These studies usually take a long period of time to conduct and are costly.

When a cohort is identified and assembled in the past on the basis of existing records and then followed to the point when the study is started, the cohort study is referred to as retrospective. In this

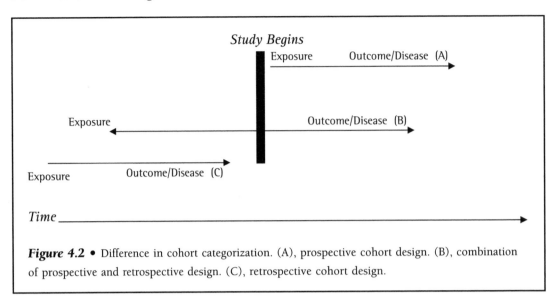

Figure 4.2 • Difference in cohort categorization. (A), prospective cohort design. (B), combination of prospective and retrospective design. (C), retrospective cohort design.

type of cohort study, both the exposure and outcome have occurred at the start of the study. The terms historical or nonconcurrent cohort study are used interchangeably with respect to retrospective cohort studies. An advantage of retrospective cohort studies is that they are less expensive and can be conducted more expeditiously than prospective studies. Use of the retrospective cohort design is also advantageous in instances when records can be linked to other registries and public information data sources. An example is occupational epidemiology, where occupational or work records can be linked to mortality and cancer registries.[7] A major disadvantage of retrospective cohort studies is the dependence on information collected prior to the planning of the study. Therefore the quality of exposure or outcome data is sometimes not the most appropriate for addressing the research questions posed.

Designs representing a combination of prospective and retrospective cohorts have been constructed and utilized. Hennekens and Buring[4] describe this mixture of prospective and retrospective cohort as occurring in ambidirection, meaning the data are collected on a cohort of subjects both prior to and following an exposure of interest. The advantage of this type of hybrid cohort study design is its ability to explore both the possible short- and long-term effects of an exposure. Cohort designs can also be altered by nesting a case-control design within the study. Information concerning an exposure or intervention is initially collected on all members of the cohort but not evaluated or studied until a later time when an appropriate number of cases have developed. At that time, the initial exposure data for both cases and controls, which are selected from the cohort, is evaluated. The advantage with this design is that it is often less costly compared to general cohort studies, especially when dealing with expensive evaluative tests. Hippisley-Cox and Coupland used a nested case-control design within a cohort study to assess the effect of drug combinations on survival in high risk patients with ischemic heart disease.[8] The nested case-control analysis was used within the context of an on-going prospective cohort design that incorporated data on over 1 million patients receiving care in 89 general practice sites within the United Kingdom.

Assessment of the appropriate choice of either a prospective or retrospective design in a study depends on a number of factors, including time and financial commitment, length of time from exposure to disease manifestation, and data source. Retrospective studies tend to require a shorter time commitment and are less expensive to complete compared to prospective studies. They also tend to be better suited for the assessment of diseases with long time periods between exposure and manifestation. Many times, retrospective cohort studies identify exposures that have occurred many years before the study begins and therefore have to utilize data sources developed for purposes other than the issue being explored or hypothesis being tested.

Strengths and Limitations

Cohort studies have a number of strengths that should be considered (Table 4.2). They are especially well-suited to assess associations when rare exposures are of interest. With the exposure as the focus, identifying rare exposures is easier than with a case control design and the opportunity to examine multiple exposures and or effects is available. Because participants are disease-free when their exposure status is defined, the temporal sequence between exposure and outcome is more obvious. Selection bias tends to have a minimal affect on cohort studies since the outcome is unknown when the exposure status is determined. Therefore, the ascertainment of exposure status is not affected by knowledge of outcome status.

However, misclassification regarding exposure status does occur leading to misclassification bias (see discussion below). Several other forms of bias that are of concern with cohort studies include loss to follow-up, interviewer/examiner objectivity, and nonparticipation bias. Of the different types of cohort studies, selection bias affects prospective cohort studies least.

Other limitations are also a factor in conducting and evaluating cohort studies. The large numbers of participants required to conduct cohort studies can lead to issues with study population identification and follow-up. Additionally, the time and financial commitments involved tend to be large. Follow-up may take years and may be very expensive to conduct.

Table 4.2
Strengths and Limitations of Case-Control and Cohort Designs

Case-control designs
  Strengths
  • Quicker and less expensive than cohort or experimental studies
  • Well-suited for evaluating diseases with long latency periods
  • Optimal for evaluating rare diseases
  • Allow for examination of multiple etiologic factors for a single disease

  Limitations
  • Inefficient for the evaluation of rare exposures
  • Prone to bias, especially recall bias and selection bias
  • Do not allow for direct calculation of incidence rates
  • Temporal sequence of exposure and outcome not always known

Cohort designs
  Strengths
  • Appropriate for evaluating rare exposures
  • Temporal sequence of exposure and outcome is clear
  • Selection and recall bias is minimized
  • Allow for direct calculation of incidence rates

  Limitations
  • Time and cost tend to be greater than case-control studies
  • Subjects are lost to follow-up over the course of the study
  • Not efficient for evaluating rare diseases

Gordis[5] explains that cohort studies are warranted when there is some indication that the exposure identified may have an association with the outcome of interest. This indication may come from previous studies or observations. Cohort studies are also very useful when attrition is minimized. In summary, cohort studies are best suited for research questions that involve rare exposures or multiple exposures, when large numbers of participants, time and financial commitments are not an issue, and when greater confidence in the relationship between exposure and outcome is vital.

Bias

Both cohort and case-control studies can experience bias due to losses to follow-up. An important assumption for the calculation of the incidence rates in a cohort study is that individuals who are lost to follow-up are similar to those who remain under observation with regard to characteristics affecting the outcome of interest. Loss to follow-up bias exists when losses are differential based on exposure and outcome (disease) status. Therefore, this bias exists when individuals who are lost to follow-up are dissimilar to those who remain in the study concerning characteristics that affect the outcome, and the losses to follow-up are different in the exposed and unexposed groups. Bias due to interviewer/examiner objectivity was discussed previously. Misclassification bias exists in cohort studies, but its effect depends on whether the bias is random or nonrandom. If it is random, misclassification occurs similarly in both the exposed and unexposed groups, which may lead to underestimation of an association if one exits. In nonrandom misclassification, misclassification causes differential accuracy in information between the exposed and unexposed groups that could lead to either an underestimation or overestimation of the risk. The effect of nonrandom misclassification on the risk estimation depends on the situation and is therefore unpredictable. Bias due to nonparticipation generally does not affect the association but it may affect the ability to generalize the results beyond the study population or sample. The association between exposure and outcome would be biased only if nonparticipation is related to both exposure status and factors affecting the outcome.

Measurement of Association

Based on the analytical process involved with cohort studies, the estimation of an incidence measure for each group is obtained after ascertainment of the outcome of interest. The incidence measures are then compared as absolute differences (attributable risk) or relative differences (relative risk) in order to measure the association between exposure and outcome.

Attributable risk (AR) is one of the measures based on an absolute difference between incidence (risk) estimates. It estimates the excess risk associated with the exposure of interest. The attributable risk of experiencing the outcome is calculated by subtracting the incidence estimate in the unexposed group from the incidence estimate in the exposed group.

$$AR = I_{exp} - I_{unexp}$$

AR: Attributable risk

I_{exp}: Incidence estimate in exposed group

I_{unexp}: Incidence estimate in unexposed group

Therefore, the attributable risk represents the risk of disease that is attributable to the exposure of interest. Because the mathematical expression is a subtraction, the units of the value remain. The calculated value of absolute risk, therefore, represents the number of cases of outcome or disease within the exposed group that is attributed to the exposure. The value representing no additional risk is 0. Values above 0 indicate that a certain number of cases can be attributed to the exposure. Values below 0 would indicate that the exposure is in some way protective. Examples of alternative measures of absolute difference include percent attributable risk in exposed individuals ($\%AR_{exp}$), or Levin's Population Attributable Risk (% Pop AR). These measures are discussed in detail in Szklo.[7]

Relative differences in risk between exposed and unexposed groups are also utilized to measure an association between exposure and outcome. These differences can be expressed as relative risk (RR). The basic 2 × 2 cross-tabulation of exposure and disease in a cohort study will be used to assist in demonstrating the calculation of relative risk.

The relative risk of developing the disease is expressed as the ratio of the risk (incidence) in exposed individuals to that in unexposed and is depicted schematically in Table 4.3.

$$RR = a/(a+b) \ / \ c/(c+d)$$

In a hypothetical example shown in Table 4.4, a new drug indicated for the treatment of cardiovascular disease serves as the exposure, and liver disease serves as outcome seen in a number of patients taking the drug.

$$RR = a/(a+b) \ / \ c/(c+d)$$
$$RR = 400/ \ 20{,}000 \ / \ 100/ \ 20{,}000$$
$$= 4.0$$

Table 4.3
2 × 2 Cross-Tabulation of Exposure and Disease in a Cohort Study

Exposure	Disease	No Disease	
Present	a	b	a + b
Absent	c	d	c + d

Table 4.4
Hypothetical Example of New Cardiovascular Drug with Liver Disease Presenting as Adverse Effect

Cardiovascular Drug	Liver Disease	No Liver Disease	
Present	400	19,600	20,000
Absent	100	19,900	20,000

This calculated value of relative risk would be interpreted in the following manner: The risk of developing liver disease is four times greater in people exposed to the drug than in people not exposed to the drug.

If the relative risk is 1.0, then the incidence in the exposed population is equal to the incidence in the unexposed population; hence, no evidence of an association between exposure and disease development (outcome) exists. If the relative risk is greater than 1.0, the incidence in the exposed is greater than the incidence in the unexposed, suggesting a positive relationship between exposure and outcome; the exposed group is at greater risk of developing the disease compared to the unexposed group. If the relative risk is less than 1.0, the incidence in the exposed is less than the incidence in the unexposed, suggesting a negative relationship between exposure and outcome that could be protective. The exposed group has less of a risk of developing the disease compared to the unexposed group.

The confidence placed in the estimate of relative risk (and odds ratio for case-control studies) is determined by the confidence interval, which is the interval within which the estimate falls with a certain level of confidence. A 95% confidence interval means that the estimate is believed to fall within the stated interval with 95% confidence. If the confidence interval crosses 1.0 for relative risk or adds ratio assessment (0.0 for attributable risk), then confidence in the relationship between exposure and outcome would be low. Statistically, the result would be considered not significant. For example, if the estimate of relative risk is 1.7, and the reported 95% confidence interval is 0.8–5.4, the confidence interval crosses 1.0. We could not say with 95% confidence that the outcome is related to the exposure of interest. Conversely, if the same point estimate of relative risk of 1.7 has a 95% confidence interval if 1.1–3.7, the confidence interval does not cross 1.0. We could say with 95% confidence that the exposure is related to the outcome of interest. Statistically, the position of the confidence interval with respect to the value of 1.0 indicates that the relationship between outcome and exposure is not significant in the first example, but significant in the second example, even though the point estimate of relative risk is the same in both examples. Another interpretation is that, given a confidence interval of 0.8–5.4 (crosses 1.0), the risk of developing the outcome in the exposed group is not significantly greater than the risk of developing the outcome in the nonexposed group. However, given a confidence interval of 1.1–3.7 (does not cross 1.0), the risk of developing the outcome in the exposed group is significantly greater than the risk of developing the outcome in the nonexposed group. Additionally, the width of the interval provides information about the variability and precision of the estimated relative risk. A broad interval can be caused by high variability in the data, perhaps related to bias, or small sample size. A broad interval also implies lack of precision of the point estimate. With a broad confidence interval, the true point estimate of relative risk may be quite different than the calculated point estimate within the confidence interval. With a narrow confidence interval, the true point estimate of relative risk necessarily will be close in value to the calculated point estimate within the confidence interval.

Cohort Study Examples

The classic example of a cohort study is the Framingham Study of cardiovascular disease. The study began in 1948 with participants from Framingham, MA.[5,9] The investigators believed that the characteristics of the town's population would be an appropriate match for the issues being studied and would maximize follow-up. A 20-year follow-up period was proposed. The defined population was selected based on location of residence and other factors not related to the exposure of interest. Over time, the study population was observed to ascertain exposure status, then follow-up began to determine which subjects developed the cardiovascular outcome(s) of interest. At the start of the study, the 5,127 men and women enrolled in the study were free of cardiovascular disease. Many exposures were defined and ascertained. Outcome events were identified through follow-up consisting of examination every 2 years and daily surveillance of hospitalizations.

More recently, cohort study design has been applied in the study of drug therapy. Two areas that have utilized this type of observational study design are drug effects and utilization. Hennessy et al.[10] explored the rates of cardiac arrest and ventricular arrhythmia in patients treated for schizophrenia (exposure). Patients treated with one of four antipsychotic drugs were identified and then followed forward using data from Medicaid programs. Crabb[11] used a cohort design to track the development of pneumonia infections in person with HIV receiving the fusion inhibitor (exposure). Choo et al.[12] investigated drug utilization by studying the possible risk factors for the over-reporting of anti-hypertensive adherence.

Summary

Research design can be conceptualized as a ladder. A ladder is a tool or instrument made for the purpose of accomplishing something, typically, reaching some height that was not possible without the ladder. The rungs of the ladder are the various research designs available to investigator and clinician. Each rung of the ladder represents a particular study design. The lower rungs represent observational study designs; the higher rungs represent experimental designs. The ladder is a continuum of confidence, cost, and time. The further up the ladder, the more time consuming and expensive the designs are. However, the further up the ladder, the more confidence one has in the results of the study, because of the design employed. The lowest rungs are case report and series, ecological, and cross sectional studies. Studies with these designs are less expensive and less time consuming to implement, but should not be the sole source of information determining clinical behavior. These lower rungs are necessary, however, in that they may provide new information and a justification to examine the proposed relationship more rigorously with an advanced design. In effect, the lower rungs are necessary to climb higher. A major improvement in designs as you rise on the ladder is the rung represented by case-control and cohort studies. This advance is due to the presence of a control group which provides the opportunity for greater internal validity. The last significant improvement along the ladder is the introduction of randomization, which introduces experimental designs.

Researchers and clinicians are encouraged to use the ladder of research design to reduce the noise-to-message ratio in their reading of the professional literature.

References

1. Shenk, D. *Data Smog*. San Francisco, CA: HarperEdge; 1997.
2. Arndt KA. Information excess in medicine: overview, relevance to dermatology, and strategies for coping. *Archiv Dermatol*. 1992;128:1249–1256.
3. Davidoff F, Haynes B, Sackett D, Smith R. Evidence based medicine. *Br Med J*. 1995; 310:1085–1086.
4. Hennekens MD, Buring JE. *Epidemiology in Medicine*. Boston, MA: Little, Brown and Company; 1987.
5. Gordis L. *Epidemiology*. 2nd ed. Philadelphia: W.B. Saunders Company; 2000.
6. Rothman KJ, *Epidemiology: An Introduction*. New York: Oxford University Press; 2002.
7. Szklo M, Nieto FJ. *Epidemiology Beyond the Basics*. Gaithersburg, MD: Aspen Publishers, Inc.; 2000.
8. Hippisley-Cox J, Coupland C. Effect of combinations of drugs on all cause mortality in patients with ischaemic heart disease: nested case-control analysis. *Br Med J*. 2005;330(7499):1059–1063

9. Kannel WB. CHD risk factors: a Framingham Study update. *Hosp Prac.* 1990;25:93–104.
10. Hennessy S, Bilkeer WB, Knauss JS, et al. Cardiac arrest and ventricular arrhythmia in patients taking antipsychotic drugs: a cohort study using administrative data. *Br Med J.* 2002;325(7372):1070.
11. Crabb C. Clinical trials for enfuvirtide. *AIDS.* 2003;17(17):N13–N14.
12. Choo PW, Rand CS, Inui TS, et al. A cohort study of possible risk factors for over-reporting of antihypertensive adherence. *BMC Cardiovasc Dis.* 2001;1:6.

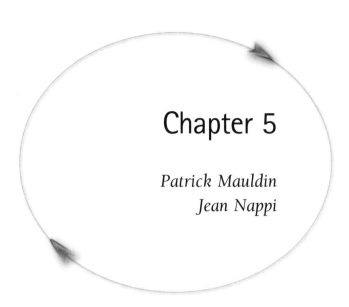

Chapter 5

Patrick Mauldin
Jean Nappi

Randomized Clinical Trials

Clinical practice guidelines are based upon evidence from clinical trials and expert opinion, and randomized clinical trials (RCTs) are widely considered to offer the best type of evidence. An RCT is a type of clinical investigation in which participants are assigned to different treatment groups by chance. This is an attempt to ensure that characteristics of the groups are similar at the initiation of the protocol. Randomization allows for better isolation of the treatment effect, with minimal influence from other factors that could affect the outcome of the study. Participants are randomly assigned to one of multiple clinical interventions, with one treatment serving as a control, and followed for a pre-specified amount of time so that a treatment effect (or outcome) can be measured. Treatment outcomes are events that occur after the participants receive one of the treatment options. Time periods for possible treatment outcomes can range from immediately following the treatment administration to months, years, or even the death of the participant, which can be many years following entry into the clinical trial. If most of the patient characteristics among the various treatment groups are similar, the true effects of the treatments can be better observed. The clear definition of endpoints, and the methods for gathering and measuring such data, must be detailed in the RCT protocol. The protocol is a document that serves as a guideline for the conduct of the trial, describing in a clear and detailed manner the endpoints, objectives, methodology, and analytical methods of the study, and serving as a historical document of the trial. Components of a standard protocol are listed in Table 5.1, with more description provided in this chapter.

Randomization

When participants are randomly allocated to treatment groups in a RCT, it means that they have a specified chance of being assigned to each treatment choice in the trial. Often the randomization scheme is set at equal chance, although sometimes this chance is 2:1 or some other unequal ratio. Randomization reduces the chance for selection bias, which could cause the experimental group to differ from the control group based on certain characteristics.[1-3] For example, selection bias might

Table 5.1
Protocol Components

- Primary and secondary objectives
- Background of disease and drug/device
- Rationale of study
- Study design, population, sites, and duration
- Inclusion/exclusion criteria
- Prohibited therapy during study
- Participant recruitment methods and screening logs
- Eligibility assessment; presentation of informed consent; randomization or registration; registration log procedure, central registration procedure, or central randomization procedure
- Baseline assessments and treatment procedures
- Drug dosage, administration, and adjustments
- Concomitant or ancillary therapy
- Clinical guidelines
- Follow-up procedure
- Notification of death
- Procedure for un-blinding

- Data collection schedule/schema
- Participant withdrawal
- Primary and secondary outcomes definitions
- Site monitoring
- Data processing, security, and confidentiality
- Data quality assurance
- Statistical considerations, sample size and power estimation, stratification, covariates, randomization, safety outcomes, missing data, interim analysis, final analysis
- Definitions of adverse event
- Regulatory and ethical obligations, informed consent, Institutional Review Board (IRB)
- Study termination, study documentation and storage, publication policy; steering committee, executive committee, and data safety and monitoring committee
- References
- Master informed consent

occur if researchers asked only a subgroup of participants in a clinical investigation to participate in a quality of life assessment. If these participants were much sicker than the average participant in the study, they would not be representative of the overall study group. Another example of selection bias might result from studying the effects of a treatment in a primarily Caucasian patient population and assuming the effect is the same for other racial groups. Selection bias may cause difficulty in the interpretation of results, as the sample participants may not be representative or able to be generalized for the intended patient population.

Various methods allow for the proper randomization of participants.[4–8] The flip of a coin could randomly allocate participants between two treatment groups in an RCT. The rule could be "heads" for treatment X and "tails" for treatment Y. Or, if more than two treatment groups are in the study, investigators could use dice, with each face (or combination of faces) of the die representing a treatment assignment. Perhaps the most common form of randomization is the use of random number generators, either from tables or computer programs. Random number generators produce a series of random numbers that are arranged in an unpredictable order. A rule is assigned for randomization, and the randomization occurs. For example, the rule could state that if the random number is odd, treatment X is assigned to the participant. However, if the number is even, the participant receives treatment Y.

Another common randomization scheme is the permuted block. This generates an allocation sequence of assignments based on a "block" of a pre-specified size being achieved.[7] For example, if the allocation ratio within a block of 20 participants was 3:1, then the block would consist of 15 X and 5 Y participants. However, the order of the entry into the block is uncertain at first. As participants are entered into the block, weight is given to achieve the pre-determined block allocation.

Many rules can be constructed for appropriate allocation of participants. If a particular characteristic or prognostic factor is important to the analysis, then stratification is a useful method for randomization. Stratification aims to balance these factors between the treatment arms of RCTs. For example, if gender is a possible prognostic factor of importance, then the treatment allocation should be balanced by an equal number of men and women in each treatment group of the study.

Trial Designs

Clinical trial designs are based on the clinical research question of interest. There are four phases of clinical trials (Figure 5.1).[1] Phase I studies are designed to assess the metabolism, absorption, toxicity, and pharmacological effects of a new drug in human studies. Participants of Phase I studies typically include healthy volunteers, and side effects are monitored to see if they are related to increasing dosage.

	I	II	III	IV
Purpose	Pharmacology	Feasibility/Efficacy	Relative Efficacy	Post-Marketing
Typical Number of Subjects	20–80	100–300	200–1000's	200–1000's

Time →

Figure 5.1 • Phases of clinical trials.

Phase II studies are clinical studies designed to test the safety and efficacy in a larger population of patients who have the disease that the drug was designed to treat. Once some pharmacologic activity has been evaluated from the results of the Phase I study, and safety as well as efficacy of the experimental treatment is observed in Phase II, Phase III studies are conducted on larger populations of sick patients, typically comparing the new treatment to the standard therapy currently used for the disease in question. Information from Phase III trials provides a basis for FDA approval. Phase IV studies are conducted following FDA approval of the drug or device and are considered postmarketing studies, to gain further information on the treatment's effect within various populations and to assess side effects, benefits, and optimal administration associated with long-term use. Phase III trials are usually randomized; on occasion Phase II trials may also be randomized when a control group is needed, particularly for critical diseases such as AIDS[9] or cancer.[10]

Randomized trials are designed as either parallel or crossover studies.[2,11] With standard parallel designs, participants receive only one of the possible treatments. For example, if a patient is randomized to treatment X, then it will be the only treatment this participant receives during the course of the trial. A similar group would receive a different therapy, and the outcomes of the two groups would be compared.

A crossover design lets each participant receive both available treatments at different time periods, separated by a washout period between the treatments.[1,12] This allows for the estimation of the within-patient treatment difference. The main advantages of crossover designs are that they (1) will not hinder recruitment, as all participants will receive each study treatment, and (2) can increase accuracy as each participant serves as his or her own control.

However, care should be taken with the design and interpretation of a crossover trial.[12,13] There may be a "carryover effect" of the first treatment that may influence the second treatment. For example, if the first treatment significantly alters the state of (or even cures) the disease in the participant before the second treatment is administered, then the treatment effect will be skewed. Often in a crossover trial one half the patients receive treatment X first, and the other half receive treatment Y first. Proper planning and statistical design should ensure a true assessment of the treatment effect from each alternative therapy. As stated previously, the design choice is based on the question being asked. It is important that the objectives be clearly defined ahead of time to ensure the most appropriate design.

Blinding

If the participant or clinician is aware of the randomized treatment assignment of the participant, a bias could occur if actions taken by either party, even unknowingly, influence the true treatment effect. For example, if the participant knows that he or she has been randomized to active medical therapy for blood pressure management rather than placebo, the participant may not adhere to the scheduled exercise and diet recommendations as closely as he or she would if assigned to the placebo arm of the trial. Similarly, a clinician overseeing his treatment may not emphasize exercise and diet factors as heavily if he or she knows the patient is receiving the treatment. Blinding keeps the treatment assignment unknown to the various parties of the RCT. If only the participants are kept unaware of the treatment assignment, this is referred to as single blind. However, if the investigators, participants, and biostatisticians evaluating the endpoints are all kept unaware, this is considered double blinding. Another type of blind, called partial blinding, allows for the identification of study participants by their treatment group without revealing the treatment by name. For example, participants will be listed as being in Group X or Y, but whether X (or Y) is the experimental treatment or control is unknown. This format is commonly used for data reports to the Data Safety and Monitoring Committee (explained below).

Individuals whose conduct could affect the interpretation of the results or the results themselves should be blinded as necessary.[14] Many factors could allow for the accidental unblinding of a study participant. These include pill appearance, packaging, treatment side effects, and patient appearance (i.e., surgical scars). Careful attention should be given with the planning of the RCT to avoid these disclosures. In addition, circumstances and methods for planned or emergent unblinding should be clearly described in the study protocol.

Endpoints

Clinical trial endpoints are the measurements that allow for the study hypotheses to be tested, and they can be either quantitative or qualitative in nature. Depending on the underlying clinical issue, examples of clinical endpoints include the improvement in symptoms, presence or absence of disease, changes in quality of life or resource utilization (i.e., costs), and time-to-event endpoints such as tumor progression, repeat hospitalizations, or death. Ideal endpoints should be clinically relevant and should clearly reflect the study objectives.[15] In addition, endpoints should be both valid and reliable. Validity assures that the endpoint you are measuring truly reflects the relevant treatment effect. Reliability addresses the extent to which the measurement obtained is reproducible; it is a measure of the random-ness of the measurement process itself. Endpoints should be capable of being accurately measured regardless of the treatment assignment, and they should be void of bias.

Endpoints can be quantified as continuous, categorical, or time-to-event. Continuous outcomes include variables that are measured on a continuous scale, such as blood pressure, number of colon polyps, weight, or lipid levels. For example, to assess the effectiveness of a daily treatment of drug X on multiple sclerosis, an appropriate endpoint would be the change in the mean number of lesions seen on pre- and post- treatment MRIs. Categorical endpoints are typically measured as success/failure or the qualitative grouping of endpoints such as scale scores. These scores are often ordinal endpoints; examples include angina class (rated from I to IV, reflecting the degree of chest pain), cancer stage (rated from I to IV reflecting the progression of cancer), and number of vision lines lost (for macular degeneration). Unfortunately, the changes from one category to another are often not necessarily scaled equal; i.e., a change from categories I to II may not equal the change from categories II to III. Finally, time-to-event endpoints are appropriate when analyzing overall survival, tumor progression, or time to relapse. For example, if the protocol assesses the efficacy of a particular treatment on participants with advanced esophageal cancer, an appropriate endpoint would be time to dysphagia relapse.

When a defined endpoint cannot be measured (for clinical or possibly financial reasons), a surrogate endpoint can be substituted.[16] A surrogate endpoint is used as a proxy for the "true" or final biological or clinical outcome. Examples include the number of MRI lesions for progression of multiple sclerosis or prostate specific antigen (PSA) for prostate cancer. The benefits of surrogate endpoints include earlier measurement and increased frequency of observations as well as an independence from potential covariates likely to affect the true endpoint.[17] The surrogate must yield a predictive ability for the clinical outcome in question and be responsive to the treatment alternatives in the RCT.[18] However, care should be taken with the use of surrogates.[19] Each surrogate endpoint requires validation to ensure appropriate measurement. As quoted in Senn, "the difference between a surrogate endpoint and a true endpoint is like the difference between a check and cash. You may get a check earlier, but it may bounce."[16]

Measurement of a surrogate endpoint may be clinically misleading. For example, prior to 1989, the efficacy of antiarrhythmic agents was usually determined by the drug's ability to suppress premature ventricular complexes (PVCs). The design of the Cardiac Arrhythmia Suppression Trial (CAST) included a placebo arm and used mortality as an endpoint.[20] In CAST, patients that received drugs that were known to decrease PVCs had a higher mortality rate than those patients randomized to placebo. Even though the drugs decreased the number of PVCs, they did not result in a better patient outcome. In this scenario, reduction of PVCs (the surrogate endpoint) was not a good measure for long-term survival.

Sample Size and Power

Sample size calculations vary depending on trial factors such as study design, patient population, and type of endpoint. There are generally four components to a sample size calculation: (1) Type II error (false-negative rate), which occurs when one fails to reject the null hypothesis when the alternative hypothesis is true (for determination of power); (2) Type I error (false-positive rate), which occurs when one falsely rejects the null hypothesis when it is true; (3) clinically relevant difference; and (4) the variance within each group.[21] With these four components pre-specified, a standard sample size calculation can be made to estimate how many patients should be enrolled into each arm of the trial to ensure a specific significance level at a specific level of power.

As mentioned earlier, clinical trial endpoints are the quantitative or qualitative measurements that correspond to the study objectives. The basic goal of any RCT protocol is to make sure there is sufficient statistical power so that proper interpretation of the endpoints can occur. Power is the probability of detecting a treatment effect if indeed there is one. Under traditional superiority testing, the null hypothesis assumes there is no difference between groups. If you reject the null hypothesis based on a certain significance level (often 0.05), then you are accepting the alternative hypothesis that there is a difference between the groups. A Type II error (false-negative rate) is defined as (1 − power). Thus, the smaller the false-negative rate, the higher the power of the study. In addition, the larger the sample size, then the higher the power, or the higher the probability of detecting a difference if it truly exists. Although there are no rigid guidelines, most prospective RCTs seek to achieve a power of at least 80% (i.e., a 20% chance of failing to reject the null when the alternative is true).

Sample size calculations should be inflated to account for unforeseen circumstances. Depending on the illness or follow-up period, participants can be lost to follow-up or may voluntarily withdraw from the study. Should either of these circumstances occur, an adequate sample of participants might not be available at the end of the study to achieve the expected power. Thus, depending on the type of illness, study design, or the experience of the investigator or clinical center with these types of clinical trials, an appropriate inflation factor should be considered for the final estimation of sample size.

Participant Recruitment

Recruitment strategies to enroll patients into RCTs should be free from any actions that may be interpreted as intimidation or persuasion.[22] Unless justified in the protocol, recruitment should be open to all patients without regard to age, gender, or ethnic characteristics (it should be noted that specific considerations are required to evaluate certain populations such as pregnant women, human fetuses, and neonates (45 CFR 46 Subpart B), prisoners (45 CFR 46 Subpart C) and children (45 CFR 46 Subpart D).[23] The objective in RCTs is to recruit participants that will adhere to the protocol requirements.[24] During the assessment of potential participants, the study investigator must provide a detailed and understandable presentation of the protocol so that a fully informed decision can be made by the potential participant to agree to the protocol requirements. Patients with a high probability of noncompliance (for reasons such as difficulties returning to the clinical center due to large geographic distances, development of a new clinical condition, or an inability to read and/or complete the self-administered forms) should not be entered into the RCT. The clinical investigator must thoroughly assess patients' understanding of the protocol and provide an atmosphere that encourages ongoing compliance.[25]

If, for any reason, a participant chooses to voluntarily withdraw from the RCT, he or she has the right to do so without influencing his or her future medical care. For participants who withdraw consent (explained below), documentation should be provided that states the date and reason for consent withdrawal, and their data should be included in the analysis up to that point in time. For participants who do not withdraw consent yet miss some clinic visits or fail to complete forms, documentation should be made for the missing data, and the participants should continue to be followed according to protocol requirements. All follow-up data for these participants should be included in the analysis.

Informed Consent

Informed consent is a process of communication between the clinical investigator and patient that ensures the complete understanding of the RCT (including risks, costs, and other treatment options), allowing the potential participant to make an informed decision as to whether or not he or she wishes to participate. The purpose of informed consent is for the patient to be an informed participant in his or her health care decisions. Patients must be considered competent to understand and process the information so that they can make an appropriate decision, and the consent must be voluntary and in accordance with U.S. FDA regulations (21 CFR 50) and guidelines.[22] The investigator must obtain consent from the participant or the participant's legally authorized representative following a thorough explanation of the purpose, potential benefits, risks, and responsibilities of the study. No RCT screening procedures should be performed for the purpose of research until consent has been obtained. All questions regarding therapy and the protocol should be answered and clearly understood prior to signing the consent, and an observer should witness the informed consent process.

Statistical Analysis Populations

In order to minimize bias in the analysis of data, a statistical plan should be devised prior to looking at the data.[26] The plan should include the rules to decide which data will be excluded from the planned statistical analysis, including ways of dealing with missing outcome and covariate data. Components in the statistical plan are listed in Table 5.2.

Typically, RCTs are designed utilizing the "intent-to-treat" principle.[27,28] This means that following randomization to a specific treatment group, each participant's data should be included in the primary analysis regardless of compliance with the protocol-specified intervention or follow-up requirements. In addition to intent-to-treat, investigators may want to assess the treatment effect when participants are compliant with protocol procedures. For example, an investigator may be interested in evaluating the treatment effect for participants who took the intervention as assigned. This type of analysis is referred to as *per protocol*. Per protocol analyses should be conducted secondary to intent-to-treat analyses for RCTs. If conclusions are the same for both analyses, then the interpretation of study results is strengthened. If there is a discrepancy, reasons for the difference can be explored. However, it is the intent-to-treat analyses that support the primary hypothesis. Intent-to-treat reduces or avoids biases (such as selection bias) that may result from excluding randomized participants who are not compliant with the protocol.

Table 5.2
Components of a Statistical Plan

- Definition of target population and study samples (target population, intent-to-treat sample, per treated sample, per protocol sample)
- General statistical considerations (patient accountability, randomization and blinding, missing data, treatment group, comparability at baseline and study conclusion, preliminary analysis, site effects, patient compliance)
- Efficacy analyses
  1. *Primary outcome variable(s)* parameter description, handling of missing outcome and covariate data, statistical hypotheses, interim analysis method, final analysis method, additional analyses
  2. *Secondary outcome variable(s)* description of analysis methods for categorical variables, continuous variables, and time to event variables

- Safety analyses (overview, definition and categorization of adverse events, descriptive statistics of adverse events, inferential statistics of adverse events, description of laboratory measures, descriptive statistics of laboratory measures, inferential statistics of adverse events, and other safety variables)
- Data to be excluded from analysis

Multicenter Trials

A high priority of all RCTs is the rapid and appropriate recruitment of participants into the clinical trial. If meeting the recruitment target is improbable by screening patients from only one clinical center, then more sites may be necessary. The necessity of multiple sites may be attributed to the fact that the clinical condition under investigation is relatively rare, and one site cannot screen enough patients to achieve targeted enrollment.[29] Similarly, if the investigator or sponsor desires a very rapid recruitment of participants into the trial for FDA approval of their drug or device, or if the trial is a large screening study that requires a very large number of participants to test the hypothesis, an RCT involving several centers may be desired. Whatever the reason, opening the trial to more than one center may increase the speed of recruitment and generalizability of the results, at a potential cost of added complexity.[16] Ensuring adherence to the protocol from geographically dispersed locations, different hospital types (public or private), or even different countries and cultures requires very careful management and oversight of the study. A strong organizational infrastructure must be in place so that appropriate protocol, ethical, financial, and data management issues can be addressed with expedience.

In RCTs, particularly multicenter RCTs, the coordinating center (CC) has the responsibility for all aspects of the day-to-day conduct of the clinical trial.[30] From the preparation of the operations manual and data collection instruments to the collection of data and final statistical analysis, the CC assumes the primary role in assisting the clinical centers with the appropriate implementation and conduct of the RCT. For multicenter RCTs, central randomization is usually performed at the CC. Central randomization provides a central location to which all screening and randomization data is sent so that the CC can allocate the randomization assignments to each clinical center participating in the RCT, providing better control of the randomization process. Centralized data management at the CC provides consistent data queries and clarifications as well as proper storage and management of all case data collection instruments. The CC has the responsibility of coordinating the central medical review and overseeing quality assurance, including regular site visits to clinical centers. Finally, given the centralized data management and project coordination, it is most efficient for the statistical responsibilities to reside with the CC. Having biostatisticians involved with each aspect of the RCT, from the protocol and forms design to the final analysis and report generation, saves time and resources and ensures that all clinical and scientific questions are answered with appropriate statistical methods.

Institutional Review Board

In accordance with U.S. FDA regulations (21 CFR 56) and guidelines, all research involving human subjects and changes to the research plan must be reviewed and approved by an institutional review board (IRB).[22] A copy of the protocol, proposed informed consent form, other written participant information, and any proposed advertising material, must be submitted to the clinical center's IRB for written approval. Before recruitment of participants, the investigator must receive a copy of the IRB approval of the protocol and informed consent form. If amendments to the protocol are ever made following the initiation of the study, the investigator must submit all protocol amendments and revisions to the informed consent document to the IRB for approval. IRB approval must be received before the amendment can be implemented. Furthermore, IRB protocol renewals must be received annually.

Adverse Events

Because the safety of participants during an RCT is of primary importance, the detailed monitoring of adverse events is required.[22] An adverse event is a serious or more prevalent event occurring during a research study that may be related to trial participation. Adverse events may involve drugs, biologics, devices, loss of confidentiality, privacy issues, or harm to others. "An adverse event can therefore be any unfavorable and unintended sign (including an abnormal laboratory finding), symptom, or disease temporally associated with the use of a medicinal (investigational) product, whether or not related to the medicinal (investigational) product."[22]

Serious adverse events (SAEs) include "any adverse therapeutic experience occurring at any dose (if a drug) that results in any of the following outcomes: death, a life-threatening adverse drug experience, inpatient hospitalization or prolongation of existing hospitalization, a persistent or significant disability/incapacity, or a congenital anomaly/birth defect."[22] Other important medical events may be considered serious adverse drug experiences if they jeopardize the patient and require medical or surgical intervention to prevent death or hospitalization.

The data safety monitoring committee (DSMC, or data safety monitoring board [DSMB]) meets on a periodic basis to review all interim data relating to the RCT.[26] The DSMC typically consists of at least three members external to the conduct of the study with expertise in RCT methodology, epidemiology, ethics, quality-of-life evaluation for clinical trials of this nature, and clinical treatments for the types of patients under investigation. The study biostatistician can participate in the DSMC meetings as a nonvoting member. The functions of the DSMC include: (1) review all adverse effects or complications related to the trial interventions, (2) review interim data on the primary and secondary outcomes according to pre-specified guidelines, (3) monitor participant enrollment, (4) review the compliance of clinical centers, and (5) recommend to the investigators and/or sponsor whether the RCT should continue as usual, be modified, or stopped. In general, clinical investigators are not present at the "closed sessions" of the DSMC but may on occasion be requested to present or provide information to assist the DSMC in carrying out its functions appropriately.

Summary

If designed and implemented appropriately, RCTs provide the strongest type of data from which clinical practice guidelines derive their recommendations. Efforts must be made to avoid bias in all steps of the process, including recruitment, randomization, treatment, and analysis. Trial design and mathematical requirements for needed statistical analysis determine the number of subjects needed for the study. Once the appropriate study design has been determined, the investigator must abide by the regulations designed to protect the human subjects who will participate. Successful research requires careful consideration of study design before embarking on the endeavor.

References

1. Piantadosi S. *Clinical Trials: A Methodologic Perspective.* New York: Wiley; 1997.
2. Rosenberger WF, Lachin JM. *Randomization in Clinical Trials: Theory and Practice.* New York: Wiley; 2002.
3. Schechtman KB. Clinical trials. In Chung-Chow S, ed. *Encyclopedia of Biopharmaceutical Statistics.* New York: Marcel Dekker; 2000.
4. Jadad AR. *Randomized Controlled Trials.* London: BMJ Publishing Group; 1998.
5. Lachin JM. Properties of simple randomization in clinical trials. *Control Clin Trials.* 1988;9:312–326.
6. Lachin JM. Statistical properties of randomization in clinical trials. *Controlled Clinical Trials.* 1988b;9:289–311.
7. Matts JP, Lachin JM. Properties of permuted-block randomization in clinical trials. *Controlled Clinical Trials.* 1988;9:327–344.
8. Zelen M. The randomization and stratification of patients to clinical trials. *J Chron Dis.* 1974;27:365–375.
9. U.S. Public Health Service. *AIDS Clinical Trials Information Service* 1997. Available: http://www.actis.org/.
10. National Institutes of Health (NIH) / National Cancer Institute, 2005: http://cancertrials.nci.nih.gov/clinicaltrials.
11. Lachin JM, Matts JP, Wei LJ. Randomization in clinical trials: conclusions and recommendations. *Controlled Clinical Trials.* 1988;9:365–374.
12. Cleophas TJM, Tavenir P. Clinical trials in chronic diseases. *J Clin Pharm.* 1995;35:594–598.
13. Jones B, Donev AN. Modeling the design of cross-over trials. *Stat Med.* 1996;15:1435–1446.
14. Day SJ, Altman DG. Statistics notes: blinding in clinical trials and other studies. *Br Med J.* 2000;321(7259):504.
15. Terrin ML. Efficient use of endpoints in clinical trials: A clinical perspective. *Stat Med.* 1990;9:155–160.
16. Senn S. *Statistical Issues in Drug Development.* New York: Wiley; 1997.
17. Herson J. The use of surrogate endpoints in clinical trials (an introduction to a series of four papers). *Stat Med.* 1989;8:403–404.
18. Prentice RL. Surrogate endpoints in clinical trials: definition and operational criteria. *Stat Med.* 1989;8:431–440.
19. Fleming TR, Demets DL. Surrogate endpoints in clinical trials: are we being misled? *Ann Intern Med.* 1996;125:605–613.
20. Cardiac Arrhythmia Suppression Trial (CAST) Investigators. Preliminary report: effect of encainide and flecainide on mortality in a randomized trial of arrhythmia suppression after myocardial infarction. *N Engl J Med.* 1989;321:406–412.
21. Lachin JM. Introduction to sample size determination and power analysis for clinical trials. *Control Clin Trials.* 1981;2:93–113.
22. Department of Health and Human Services, Food and Drug Administration. International Conference on Harmonization Good Clinical Practice (ICH GCP) Guidelines 1996. Available: http://www.fda.gov/cder/guidance/959fnl.pdf.
23. Department of Health and Human Services, Office for Human Research Protections, Title 45 of the Code of Federal Regulations, Part 46, Protection of Human Subjects, 2001. Available: http://www.hhs.gov/ohrp/humansubjects/guidance/45cfr46.htm#46.404
24. Spilker B, Cramer JA, eds. *Patient Recruitment in Clinical Trials.* New York: Raven Press; 1992.
25. Cramer JA, Spilker B, eds. *Patient Compliance in Medical Practice and Clinical Trials.* New York:

Raven Press; 1991.

26. Department of Health and Human Services, Food and Drug Administration, Statistical Principles for Clinical Trials (E9) 1998. http://www.fda.gov/cder/guidance/ICH_E9-fnl.PDF

27. Fischer LD, Dixon DO, Herson J, Frankowski RK, Hearron MS, Pearce KE. Intention-to-treat in clinical trials, in Pearce KE, ed. *Statistical Issues in Drug Research and Development.* New York: Marcel Dekker; 1990.

28. Lee YJ, Ellenberg JH, Hirtz DG, Nelson KB. Analysis of clinical trials by treatment actually received: is it really an option? *Stat Med.* 1991;10:1595–1605.

29. Huster WJ. Multicenter trials. In Chung-Chow S, ed. *Encyclopedia of Biopharmaceutical Statistics.* New York: Marcel Dekker; 2000.

30. Meinert, CL. *Clinical Trials: Design, Conduct, and Analysis.* Oxford: Oxford University Press; 1986.

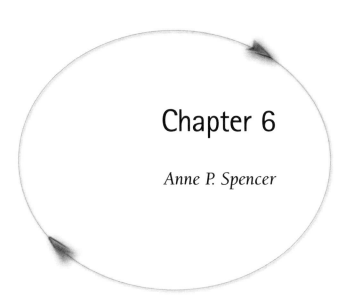

Chapter 6

Anne P. Spencer

Meta-Analysis

A meta-analysis can be viewed as a quantitative review of existing evidence. This type of assessment permits data from different, yet similar, studies to be combined and statistically analyzed. Compared to narrative reviews, meta-analyses provide an objective and quantitative assessment of available data.[1] Meta-analyses may be useful to employ when studies on the same topic individually lack substantial power, available results support different conclusions, or when a more precise estimate of treatment effect is desired.

Similar to all research endeavors, an unanswered medical question is the impetus for a meta-analysis. Sometimes, the issue has been addressed with randomized controlled trials, however some doubt remains or a discrepancy exists. In short, a meta-analysis is accomplished by identifying all studies addressing the issue, applying pre-determined criteria to select the pertinent ones, combining the data in a weighted fashion, and, finally, performing statistical analysis. Ideally, the results of a meta-analysis quantify the treatment effect size with some precision, or, conversely, provide solid support for the null hypothesis of no treatment effect.

Like any well-designed clinical study, a prospectively developed, detailed protocol is paramount for a robust and meaningful meta-analysis.[2] The specific study objectives and hypotheses tested must be detailed at the outset in order to clearly and consistently guide the process as it develops. Furthermore, criteria for study selection, data to be extracted from included studies, outcomes to be assessed, and data analysis, including subgroup analyses, should be specified in the protocol.[3]

When appropriately performed, meta-analyses may permit the realization and quantification of a treatment effect previously not detected due to inadequate power of individual studies. A small, but nonetheless important, treatment effect may require thousands of study subjects to be assessed, especially if a relatively large sampling variability exists. Individual studies rarely include this many subjects, and a meta-analysis overcomes this barrier. Similarly, a meta-analysis that confirms the null hypothesis provides assurance that lack of power was not the reason the individual studies failed to detect a treatment effect. Additionally, conflicting outcomes or outcomes of variable magnitudes may be reconciled with a well-designed meta-analysis. The meta-analysis provides a weighted contribution of effect size, so data outliers in effect or magnitude of effect are minimized, and the global treatment effect can be quantified with confidence.

Narrative reviews often address areas of controversy or conflict, however, they are subjective and prone to the bias of the authors. Appropriately performed meta-analyses are guided by rules and standards that govern which studies to include and dictate how to balance the quantitative evidence each provides.[4] Two meta-analyses addressing the same topic should yield the same result independent of the researcher performing it.

Study Eligibility and Data Search

Prior to searching for studies to be included in a meta-analysis, methods for study identification and selection must be delineated. The researcher must specify his or her search strategy, including data-bases and publications to be examined for included data. Next, parameters defining acceptable study design for inclusion must be determined. Ideally only randomized, double-blinded trials that performed intention-to-treat analyses should be included. However, deviations from this ideal may be necessary, based on the available data. It is preferable for both published and unpublished data to be included as this minimizes the effect of "publication bias." This bias reflects the influence of the nature and direction of the study results on its likelihood to be published.[4] This bias exists because published studies are not representative of all studies performed on a given subject. In general, studies with negative or neutral findings are less likely to be published than ones with positive findings.[5]

In addition to study design characteristics, study content characteristics necessary for the study to be included must also be determined. For example, suppose a meta-analysis is undertaken to assess the impact of aspirin therapy on the primary prevention of myocardial infarction. It would be important to provide characteristics of the trials to be included in the analysis, such as the patient population. Are trials including only very high-risk patients (e.g., presence of multiple risk factors, such as advanced age, hypertension, and diabetes) to be assessed, or are low-risk patient populations also to be included?

It is generally important to ensure the patient populations in the various trials are somewhat similar in order to have meaningful results. Combining data from patient populations with very different baseline rates of events (e.g., high-risk versus low-risk) can potentially render the results of the meta-analysis meaningless.

The comparison treatment also needs to be determined. To continue the aspirin example, researchers must decide whether they want to assess the effects of aspirin compared to placebo or active therapy, such as high-dose aspirin, naproxen, or some other medication. The desired comparator needs to be specified so only trials that include this medication will be included in the meta-analysis. Furthermore, the dose or dose range of aspirin to be included needs to be specified. It is likely that various aspirin dosages have been studied for the primary prevention of myocardial infarction. Specifying and limiting the dosages to be included will minimize the potential confounding effect of various dosages on both efficacy and side effects.

Similarly, the specific patient outcomes that must be assessed in a trial for it to be a part of the meta-analysis should be determined. Using the same example, one would assume the outcome of myocardial infarction would be required, however, any secondary outcomes that are to be addressed also need to be included.

See Table 6.1 for an example of the parameters that have been considered and ultimately selected in the design phase of this hypothetical meta-analysis to assess the impact of aspirin in the primary prevention of myocardial infarction. In addition to those listed and discussed here, other parameters determined to be important by the investigator that would affect the inclusion and exclusion of available trials should also be detailed. It is important for the designer of a meta-analysis to thoroughly define all pertinent characteristics prior to study selection to ensure the unbiased selection of studies and a homogenous pooled patient population. This leads to robust and clinically applicable findings.

Once the methods for study selection have been finalized, thorough searches to identify research for potential inclusion need to be performed. In order to minimize publication bias, it is essential that multiple databases be searched and all identified research meeting the stated criteria be included in analysis. Possible sources to identify studies for assessment include computerized bibliographic databases of published and unpublished research, review articles, abstracts, conference/symposia proceedings, books, granting agencies, and trial registries.[2]

Data Extraction

There are two levels of data extraction in the performance of a meta-analysis. The first involves the selection of studies from all that were identified during searches of various databases. Documentation addressing how each identified study either did or did not meet eligibility requirements must be captured. Second, for all studies deemed eligible for inclusion, relevant outcomes and other data must be abstracted.[6] The method for data abstraction must be reliable. This is best accomplished by developing a form for data collection and having at least two individuals independently abstract the data. The influence of human error can be minimized by reconciling the results obtained by the different abstractors.[6]

Data Analysis

Data are analyzed using a weighted average of the results, in which the larger trials have a greater effect than the smaller ones. Once pertinent data have been extracted from the studies, heterogeneity is

Table 6.1

Example of Study Eligibility Parameters for the Design of a Meta-Analysis to Assess Aspirin in the Primary Prevention of Myocardial Infarction

Parameter	Options*	Decision
Data source	• Published data • Published and unpublished data	Published and unpublished data
Data	• Retrospectively obtained • Prospectively randomized	Propectively randomized
Treatment status	• Unblinded • Single-blinded • Double-blinded	Double-blinded
Reporting of results	• Intention-to-treat • Per protocol	Intention-to-treat

Patient population	• Previous myocardial infarction
	  –yes
	  –no
	• Diabetes
	  –included
	  –excluded
	  –required
	• Other risk factors (e.g., family history, smoking, hypertension)
	  –any required?
	  –any excluded?
	  –require a certain number?
	• Age range
	• Gender
	  –male only
	  –female only
	  –males and females
	• Race
	  –any race(s) excluded?
	  –limit to one race or country?
	• Many others
		• No history of myocardial infarction
		• Patients must have at least one risk factor for myocardial infarction
		• Males must be > 40 years of age
		• Females must be > 50 years of age and not receiving any hormone therapy

Aspirin	75 mg daily 81 mg daily 325 mg daily 650 mg daily A dosage range?	Aspirin 75–325 mg daily
Comparator medication	Placebo High-dose aspirin Naproxen Warfarin Other antiplatelet (e.g., dipyridamole, clopidogrel, ticlopidine)	Placebo

(continued)

Table 6.1 (cont'd)
Example of Study Eligibility Parameters for the Design of a Meta-Analysis to Assess Aspirin in the Primary Prevention of Myocardial Infarction

Parameter	Options*	Decision
Outcomes	Death	• Death
	Cardiovascular death	• Myocardial infarction
	Myocardial infarction	• Ischemic stroke
	Hospitalization	• Major and minor bleeding complications
	Cardiovascular hospitalization	
	Development of heart failure	
	Ischemic stroke	
	Coronary revascularization (e.g., PCI, CABG)	
	Bleeding complication	
	–minor	
	–major	
	–minor and major	

*All possible options not listed, just the primary ones selected for consideration.

assessed, often by the X^2 distribution. When the selected trials are homogenous, a fixed-effects model is appropriate for analysis. This model assumes the variation in estimated treatment effects between studies is only due to random error.[7] Ideally, a well-designed meta-analysis, in which studies reflecting the same therapy in the same population have been selected, will yield homogenous trials.

However, at times heterogeneity is detected between studies. In this case, a random-effects model is appropriate. In contrast to the fixed-effects model, this model assumes no single true treatment effect exists, but rather that each study has a different, but true, effect. It is assumed the population of truths follows a normal distribution.[8] In general, neither fixed-effects nor random-effects models are ideal. The premise that all available studies are essentially identical seems oversimplified. Random-effects models statistically accommodate for heterogeneity; however, they shed no light on why the heterogeneity between treatment effects exists. Hopefully, each model will result in a similar pooled treatment effect; however, the random-effects model is less likely to reach statistical significance.[9]

Deeming the data included in meta-analysis as either heterogeneous or homogenous can also be viewed as oversimplification, especially as this designation is largely influenced by the number of trials included in the analysis. Meta-analyses with fewer trials are less likely to be composed of heterogeneous studies. To decrease reliance on this dichotomous designation, a relatively new term, I^2, has been developed to quantify heterogeneity between trials. I^2 can range in value between 0% and 100%. The presence of no heterogeneity is assigned a value of 0%, and larger values indicate increasing heterogeneity. I^2 is the percentage of variation across the studies that cannot be attributed to chance. In addition to statistically significant heterogeneity, the magnitude of heterogeneity can be assessed. For example, a meta-analysis including 125 trials and 150,000 study subjects may be statistically heterogeneous. But if the I^2 value is 4%, the reader can have some assurance that the magnitude of heterogeneity is minimal. Similarly, an I^2 value of 65% indicates that a lot of heterogeneity exists. Strict categorization of heterogeneity is not appropriate for all study types; however, general categorizations for consideration are low (25%), moderate (50%), and high (75%).[10] A review of over 500 meta-analyses indicate that about 25% had I^2 values of 50% or greater.[11]

Limitations

The quality of the included trials is of paramount importance, and this may be more difficult to assess in a meta-analysis than in a single prospective clinical trial. However, the importance of this aspect cannot be overemphasized. For example, a 30%–40% larger treatment effect is estimated to occur in studies that did not adequately report the presence of double-blinding versus those studies that did, potentially resulting in detection bias.[12] While the true impact of methodological design on treatment effect is unknown, it appears to be substantial. The quality of the individual studies included in a meta-analysis must be ensured to minimize the numerous types of biases that can affect individual results, such as selection bias, performance bias, detection bias, and attrition bias. For these reasons, strict criteria outlining the characteristics that must be possessed by individual studies in order to be included must be reported. The methods section of a meta-analysis should clearly delineate these characteristics. Not only is the design quality of the individual studies important, but the homogeneity between studies must also be substantial in order to yield a meaningful result. This is the most subjective aspect of conducting a meta-analysis, and it requires an investigator and a reviewer knowledgeable in both the disease state and meta-analysis techniques to assess whether patient characteristics, treatment characteristics, and treatment outcomes were appropriately included or excluded.

For example, in a meta-analysis assessing the impact of a treatment on a cardiovascular outcome, patients with diabetes should either be present or not present in all studies included. Diabetes is a tremendous risk factor for cardiovascular disease, and the baseline rate of cardiovascular events is substantially different between patients with and without diabetes. If studies with different inclusion criteria in reference to diabetes patients were combined, the baseline event rates and treatment effect rates would be substantially skewed based on this one factor. Inclusion or exclusion of this patient population in individual studies may be entirely appropriate, but the combination of data that both include and exclude this population would not be.

Example

Several studies have suggested that despite similar blood pressure control, patients treated with calcium channel blockers are at higher risk of coronary events than patients treated with other antihypertensive agents. However, no individual study was able to address this issue satisfactorily, due to the large number of events necessary to detect a relatively small between-group difference. However, even a small treatment effect difference is clinically important because of the prevalence of hypertension. A difference of only 10% could translate into thousands of excess patient events per year. In December 2000, a meta-analysis was published addressing this issue.[13] The investigators chose to include randomized controlled trials published in peer-reviewed journals that included at least 100 patients with hypertension treated with either a calcium channel blocker or another antihypertensive agent in whom cardiovascular events were assessed after a minimum of 2 years follow-up. Nine trials met the inclusion criteria, representing 27,743 patients. Patients were from the USA, Europe, Israel, and Japan. Four studies were double-blinded (30% of patients), and five were open-label. Eight trials reported intention-to-treat results (one study was missing outcome data for 4% of the participants), and one study provided per protocol results. Seven trials used dihydropyridine calcium antagonists, and two trials used verapamil or diltiazem (nondihydropyridine calcium antagonists). Various other antihypertensives, including diuretics, beta-blockers, angiotensin converting enzyme inhibitors, and clonidine were used as comparative agents. For all outcomes, a fixed-effects model was used.

The analysis concluded that use of a calcium channel blocker for hypertension versus other agents was associated with an increased odds ratio for myocardial infarction (1.26), heart failure (1.25), and the composite of major cardiovascular events (1.10). No statistically significant increases in stroke or all-cause mortality were detected. Sensitivity analyses were conducted, and when only double-blinded trials were assessed, the increased risk of myocardial infarction remained, but all other outcomes failed to reach statistical significance. Additional subgroup analyses based on the type of calcium antagonist (dihydropyridine vs. nondihydropyridine, and long-acting vs. intermediate- or short-acting), the presence of diabetes, and specific comparator antihypertensive yielded variable results for the different cardiovascular endpoints.

This meta-analysis is an example of using available data to address a concern hinted at in the medical literature. The study design can be criticized for including only published data in peer-reviewed literature (publication bias), including data from open-label trials (performance bias), and permitting trials that did not report outcomes for all patients (attrition bias). One could also argue that the various calcium channel blockers (dihydropyridine vs. nondihydropyridine, and short- vs. intermediate- or long-acting) have important inherent differences that could impact the homogeneity of this group. However, it is likely that had all of the ideal characteristics of a meta-analysis been adhered to, no studies or few studies would have met the inclusion criteria. Balancing the ideal characteristics of a meta-analysis with the need for data to analyze is a common dilemma for investigators. The performance of various subgroup analyses by the investigators was helpful. Although the major results did not change substantially, some interesting findings were reported that may be hypothesis generating for future research endeavors.

This meta-analysis is an example of one with methodological flaws, yet also representative of perhaps the best that can be done with the available data. The methods section of every meta-analysis should be thorough and detailed. This allows the reader to be aware of the shortcomings and strengths of a meta-analysis while interpreting the results.

Cumulative Meta-Analysis

Cumulative meta-analysis is the repeated performance of a meta-analysis in a chronological fashion. Essentially, an existing meta-analysis is updated with recently available data and then reanalyzed. Since lack of power often limits the occurrence of positive findings in disease states with low event rates, several studies may individually support the null hypothesis. However, once combined, the pooled sample size and treatment effect size may be adequate to generate a statistically significant finding. Figure 6.1 provides mortality results from a retrospectively performed cumulative meta-analysis of beta-blockers in secondary prevention of myocardial infarction that was published in 1999. During the late 1960s and 1970s, several studies were published addressing this issue, but none were able to provide a conclusive answer to the question: Are beta-blockers useful in the prevention of another myocardial infarction? By 1981, cumulative evidence suggested they were. However, meta-analyses were not performed at that time, and the issue was still under debate. Had a meta-analysis been performed, all available data could have been quantified, and perhaps this standard of care would have been realized at an earlier date. As additional trials were added to the model, it becomes clear that they were simply confirming the known benefits of beta-blockade after myocardial infarction.[4]

In summary, cumulative meta-analyses may be a useful tool in a prospective fashion if a clear consensus does not exist and data are continuing to be generated. The lack of consistently significant findings may be unmasked once the power shortfalls often experienced by smaller trials or disease states with low event rates are minimized by a cumulative meta-analysis.

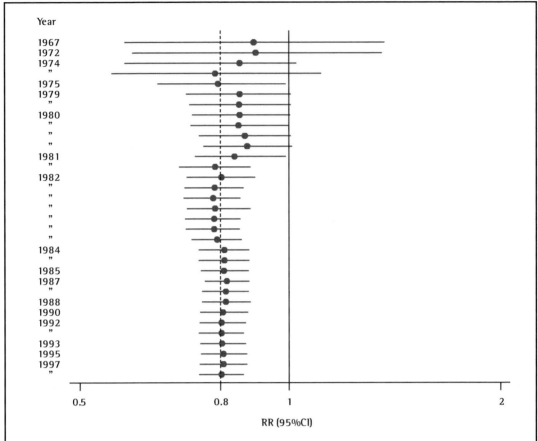

Figure 6.1 • Cumulative meta-analysis of controlled trials of beta-blockers in secondary prevention after myocardial infarction.[4]

Conclusion

Meta-analyses are useful to confirm, refute, or clarify existing evidence, especially when the power of available studies is of questionable strength and/or a small treatment effect exists. A properly executed meta-analysis will either support the null hypothesis with more conviction than previously possible, confirm a finding with increased precision, or endorse the significance of an outcome previously detected as a trend in several studies, but was not a consistently statistically significant finding.

Like all research studies, the quality of the methods is central to the quality of the results. Methods to identify and select studies, clearly specified inclusion and exclusion criteria, study design characteristics, patient populations to be included, and outcomes to be assessed must all be stated prior to data collection and analysis. Well-developed methods are most likely to lead to unbiased and homogenous data. The data abstraction methods must also be specified and should be framed to decrease bias and error. The final step, or analysis, is essentially a weighted average of the results, employing the appropriate model based on the degree of heterogeneity of the data.

Since meta-analyses are often viewed as the "final answer" or "best answer," their quality should be held to a high standard. A thorough understanding of an individual analysis' methodological strengths and limitations is paramount to one's interpretation of its estimate of effect.

References

1. Antman EM, Lau J, Kulpenick B, Mosteller F, Chalmers TC. A comparison of results of meta-analyses of randomized controlled trials and recommendations of clinical experts: treatments for myocardial infarction. *JAMA.* 1992;268:240–8.
2. Cook DJ, Sackett DL, Spitzer WO. Methodologic guidelines for systematic reviews of randomized control trials in healthcare from the Potsdam Consultation on Meta-analysis. *J Clin Epidemiol.* 1995;48:167–71.
3. Pogue J, Yusuf S. Overcoming the limitation of current meta-analysis of randomized controlled trials. *Lancet.* 1998;351:47–52.
4. Egger, M, Smith GD, Sterne JAC. Uses and abuses of meta-analysis. *Clin Med.* 2001;1:478–84.
5. Sterne JAC, Egger M, Smith GD. Investigating and dealing with publication and other biases in meta-analysis. *Br Med J.* 2001;323:101–5.
6. Petitti DB. *Meta-analysis, Decision Analysis, and Cost-effective Analysis.* 2nd ed. New York: Oxford University Press; 2000.
7. Hedges LV. Fixed effect models. In: Cooper H, Hedges LV, eds. *The Handbook of Research Synthesis.* New York: Russell Sage Foundation; 1994:285–99.
8. Raudenbush SW. Random effects models. In: Cooper H, Hedges LV, eds. *The Handbook of Research Synthesis.* New York: Russell Sage Foundation; 1994:301–21.
9. Lau J, Ioannidis JPA, Schmid CH. Summing up the evidence: one answer is not always enough. *Lancet.* 1998;351:123–7.
10. Higgins JPT, Thompson SG, Deeks JJ, Altman GD. Measuring inconsistency in meta-analyses. *Br Med J.* 2003;327:557–60.
11. Sterne JAC, Bradburn MJ, Egger M. Meta-analysis in STATA. In: Egger M, Davey Smith G, Altman DG, eds. *Systematic Reviews in Health Care: Meta-Analysis in Context.* 2nd ed. London: BMJ Publications; 2001:347–69.
12. Schulz KF, Chalmers I, Hayes RJ, Altman D. Empirical evidence of bias: dimensions of methodologic quality associated with estimates of treatment effects in controlled trials. *JAMA* 1995;273:408–12.
13. Pahor M, Psaty BM, Alderman MH, et al. Health outcomes associated with calcium antagonists compared with other first-line antihypertensive therapies: a meta-analysis of randomized controlled trials. *Lancet.* 2000;356:1949–54.

Descriptive Statistics and Univariate Analysis

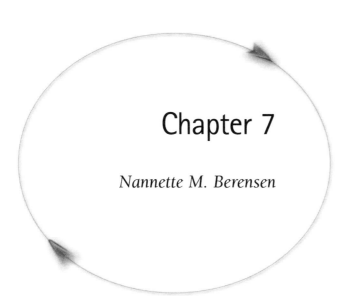

Chapter 7

Nannette M. Berensen

Statistical Tests

A basic understanding of statistics is essential to appropriately evaluate biomedical literature. When faced with therapeutic problems, practitioners frequently rely on what is published in the literature to guide them in developing the best treatment plans for their patients. Those who are involved in designing and conducting research also rely on what has already been published to direct them in designing investigations that result in new knowledge. Being a skilled user of medical literature requires the reader to make an assessment of the validity of the investigation, and this includes the statistics that were used. The clarity of data presentation and quality of statistical procedures employed are important determinants that affect the validity and resultant impact of the investigation.

The objective of this chapter is to introduce the reader to basic statistical terminology, concepts, and tests commonly used for presenting, analyzing, and interpreting information contained in research reports. It is designed for the reader with a limited knowledge of statistics. The content is intended to promote an understanding of basic statistical concepts rather than focus on computational ability. Rather than perform the work of a statistician, the goal is for readers to be able to determine whether the statistical methods used in the research reports they encounter appear to be appropriate.

Building Blocks

The purpose of statistical methods is to enable practitioners and researchers to use observations made on a subset of a population to understand the whole. This process is referred to as *estimation.* In statistics, the term *population* refers to the whole (i.e., the collection of all possible measurements that could be used to answer a study question); the term *sample* refers to a subset of members drawn from a defined population under study. It is essential that the sample be representative of the larger population of interest. Measurements that describe a population are called *parameters,* and those that are computed from a sample are referred to as *statistics.* Sample statistics are used to estimate corresponding population parameters. In general, statistics are further categorized as being *descriptive* or *inferential.* Descriptive statistics are used to summarize data into a useful form. Descriptive statistics include the measures of central tendency (e.g., mean, median, mode) and measures of variability (e.g., standard deviation, standard error of the mean, range). Inferential statistics are used to make inferences about a population from a sample. We will learn more about descriptive and inferential statistics later in the chapter. The following example will review the concepts of sample and population and introduce the concepts of randomization and selection bias.

Investigators conducted a prospective, randomized, double-blind, placebo-controlled, multicenter trial to determine the effects of ezetimibe, a cholesterol absorption inhibitor, on plasma lipids in patients with primary hypercholesterolemia.[1] The investigators enrolled 827 patients. This cohort comprised the sample, which was drawn from the population of patients with primary hypercholesterolemia. This study was described as being randomized. Random assignment means that each of the 827 patients enrolled had an equal and independent chance of being assigned to receive ezetimibe or placebo. If nonrandom assignment of these study subjects was used, the investigators may have assigned subjects with much higher plasma lipid concentrations to receive placebo and those with much lower plasma lipid concentrations to receive ezetimibe; thereby biasing the study in favor of the lipid-lowering effects of ezetimibe. The intent of randomization is to produce study groups that are similar with respect to known and unknown risk factors, to remove selection bias, and to ensure that statistical tests will have valid significance levels. It is important to note that although randomization assigns treatment groups without selection bias, it does not necessarily produce balanced groups with respect to baseline characteristics. Thus, the skilled reader knows to review the baseline demographics to assess whether the groups are similar in this regard.

There are several types of randomization: simple, blocked, and stratified. A commonly cited example of a simple randomization procedure is the coin toss; if the coin lands heads up, the subject is assigned to treatment A, if the coin lands tails up, the subject is assigned to treatment B. A disadvantage of using simple randomization is that at any given point in time, including the end of the study, the groups may be unequal in size. This disparity in group size translates into a decreased ability to detect true differences between groups. Therefore, it is more common for a blocked randomization scheme to be used.

Blocked randomization, also known as permuted block randomization, is used to ensure that at any given point in time the groups will be similar or equal in size. In the blocked randomization method, a block size is selected (e.g., four, six, or eight). If a block size of four is selected and there are two treatment groups, assuming a 1:1 patient assignment, for each block of 4 patients enrolled, two patients would be randomized to treatment A and two patients would be randomized to treatment B. The order of how the patients are assigned is random based on the possible arrangements. For example, using a block size of four, there are six possible arrangements (i.e., ABAB, BABA, AABB, ABBA, BBAA, and BAAB). One of these arrangements is selected randomly and assignment to the specified group is made accordingly. This procedure is repeated as needed until randomization is complete.

There are instances when certain characteristics of the sample can confound the results of a trial. A confounding variable is a characteristic or factor that is unequally distributed between the treatment and control groups and which also affects the outcome of interest. For example, if investigators are interested in determining whether bucindolol reduces mortality in patients with advanced heart failure, the composition of the groups studied with respect to disease severity is important. If a disproportionate number of patients randomized to receive bucindolol were New York Heart Association functional class IV patients who had much lower ejection fractions compared with those randomized to placebo who were predominately New York Heart Association functional class III patients who had better cardiac ejection fractions, the results may suggest an increased mortality rate associated with bucindolol. In fact, it is more likely that the increased mortality is associated with the patients' lower cardiac ejection fractions and more advanced disease. In this example, the differences among the bucindolol-treated patients and the placebo-treated patients may be due to confounding variables, disease severity and cardiac ejection fraction. To avoid this problem, the population of interest (i.e., those with advanced heart failure) is separated into nonoverlapping groups, called *strata*, based on key patient characteristics. Then a random sample is selected from each stratum. This would be referred to as a stratified, random sample. Investigators use stratification when a specific factor or factors (e.g., sex, race, disease severity, smoking status) can confound the study outcomes of interest.

Descriptive Statistics

Measures of Central Tendency

Descriptive statistics should provide an unbiased, complete, and summarized view of the data obtained. Descriptive statistics include the measures of central tendency (e.g., mean, median, mode) and measures of variability.

The mean is the arithmetic average of individual data points (i.e., the sum of all data points divided by the number of data points). The reader is referred to the *Types of Data* section for a definitions of continuous, ordinal, and nominal data. The mean is useful for describing continuous data. Calculating the mean for ordinal data is misleading and invalid, because the distance between numeric units is not equal. In addition, the mean is extremely sensitive to outliers. To illustrate this point consider the information in Table 7.1. Notice that each data set is comprised of five data points. Changing just one data point in data set B compared with data set A resulted in a greater than 7-fold increase in the mean.

The median is the value above (or below) which half of the data points fall. It is the 50th percentile value of a distribution, and the median is not sensitive to outliers. To illustrate this point, look again at the above example; in both data sets the median value is 3. The median in the second data set was unaffected by the value of the outlier (i.e., data point that equaled 100). The median is more useful than the mean to describe data when outliers are present or when continuous data are not normally distributed. The definition of a normal distribution is in the Presentation of Data section. A median may be used to describe continuous or ordinal data.

Table 7.1
Data Sets A, B, and C

Data Set	Data Points	Sum of Data Points	Computation of Mean	Mean ($\overline{X}$)	Median	Mode
A	1, 2, 3, 4, 5	15	15/5	3	3	–
B	1, 2, 3, 4, 100	110	110/5	22	3	–
C	1, 2, 2, 2, 3	10	10/5	2	2	2

The mode is the most commonly obtained value in the distribution. The mode is useful to describe nominal, ordinal, or continuous data. The mode for data set C is 2.

Measures of Variability

Measures of variability allow the investigator or reader to assess the variability or spread of the data. Measures of variability include the range, interquartile range, standard deviation, and standard error of the mean. The range is the difference between the largest and the smallest values in the distribution. Because the range is computed based on the lowest and highest values in a distribution, the presence of one outlier can have a tremendous impact on the range.

The interquartile range is a measure of variability directly related to the median. Interquartile range is described by the interval between the 25th and 75th percentile values. It should be used to describe the variability for ordinal data. The interquartile range clearly defines where the middle 50% of measures occur and also indicates the spread of the data.

The standard deviation (SD) is the most commonly used estimate of variability. It measures the spread of individual measurements about the sample mean. The SD is meaningful only when it is calculated for normally or near-normally distributed, continuous data. It is appropriate for describing the subject-to-subject variation within a data set. SD is computed by taking the square root of the variance. Recall that in a normal distribution, 68% of the data points fall within ± 1 SD of the mean ($\overline{X}$), 95% of the data points fall within ± 2 SD of the mean, and 99.7% of the data points fall within ± 3 SD of the mean. For example, investigators measured systolic blood pressure (SBP) on 100 first-year pharmacy students who were randomly selected. The mean SBP was computed to be 110 mmHg, and the SD computed to be 10 mmHg. From this information, it is correct to assume that 95 of the first-year pharmacy students included in the sample had SBPs between 90 mmHg and 130 mmHg; whereas, 5 had SBPs that were either less than 90 mmHg or greater than 130 mmHg.

The standard error of the mean (SEM) is a statistic computed from the SD. Mathematically, it is equal to SD divided by the square root of n; where n is the number of subjects in the sample (SEM = SD / $\sqrt{n}$). By looking at the equation for SEM, it is apparent that SEM is always smaller than the SD, except for the case when n = 1. Furthermore, it is apparent that the standard error decreases as the sample size increases, and it increases as the SD increases. From the example above, the SEM equals 1 mmHg (SEM = SD /$\sqrt{n}$ = 10 / $\sqrt{100}$). The SEM is useful for describing the sample-to-sample variability among all possible sample means. It is useful for describing how precisely the computed sample mean estimates the true, but unmeasured, mean in the larger population of interest. For example, assume the experiment of measuring SBPs on 100 first-year pharmacy students was repeated several times. The samples for each experiment would again be randomly selected from the larger population of interest (i.e., all first-year pharmacy students). Each time the experiment is performed, a different mean SBP would likely be obtained, because each sample would be comprised of different students (see Table 7.2).

Table 7.2
Results from Repeating SBP Experiment in
100 First-Year Pharmacy Students

Sample ($n = 100$)	Mean ($\overline{X}$) SBP (mmHg)
1	110
2	111
3	112
4	109
5	114

The SEM is a measure of the precision with which a single sample mean estimates the true, but unmeasured, mean in the larger population of interest. The smaller the value of the SEM, the more confident the investigator or reader is about making inferences about what the true, but unmeasured, mean value would be in the larger population of interest. SEM quantifies the uncertainty in the estimate of the mean obtained.

It is not uncommon for investigators to report their findings as a point estimate +/- SEM rather than as ± SD. This is often purposeful to make the data appear to have less variation. If readers fail to recognize this important difference, they may be misled. For example, a meta-analysis of double-blind, placebo-controlled trials was conducted to test the hypothesis that relatively small, long-term weight loss significantly improves glucose tolerance and reduces the rate of diabetes onset in obese subjects.[2] The mean weight loss in the orlistat group was reported as 6.72 kg ± SEM = 0.41 kg, and the mean weight loss reported in the placebo-treated group was 3.79 kg ± SEM = 0.38 kg. However, when you compute the SD using the SEM and sample size for the orlistat- and placebo-treated patients, the results look quite different (i.e., mean weight loss orlistat-treated group, 6.72 kg ± SD = 7.77 kg; mean weight loss placebo-treated group, 3.79 kg ± SD 6.79 kg). Thus, the mean weight change in 95% of the patients treated with orlistat ranged from a gain of 8.82 kg to a loss of 22.25 kg; whereas, the mean weight change in 95% of the patients treated with placebo ranged from a gain of 9.73 kg to a loss of 17.31 kg. When comparing mean weight loss between the two groups ± SEM, orlistat looks much better than placebo, and the two groups' SEMs are similar. However, when you evaluate the data using SD, the results aren't quite as striking.

Presentation of Data

A frequency distribution is a graph that demonstrates the number of times a particular measurement was obtained within the sample being studied. As such, frequency distributions vary in shape and size depending on what was measured. A normal or Gaussian distribution is shown in Figure 7.1.

Notice that the normal distribution is symmetric and bell-shaped about the mean ($\overline{X}$), which is also equal to the median and mode. In a normal distribution, 68% of the data points fall within ± 1 SD of the mean ($\overline{X}$), 95% of the data points fall within ± 2 SD of the mean, and 99.7% of the data points fall within ± 3 SD of the mean.

A bimodal distribution has two peaks that represent the areas of data clustering. In a bimodal distribution, the mean may be equal to the median; however, neither provides an adequate representation of the data. For example, 100 subjects were weighed. There were 50 females and 50 males. The mean and median were computed and equaled 75 kg. However, after closer evaluation, you

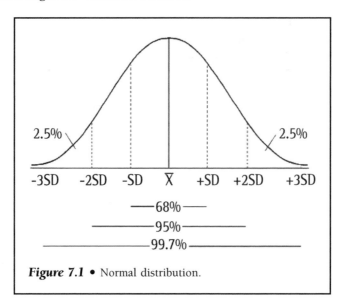

Figure 7.1 • Normal distribution.

see that the first peak represents the body weights of the females and the second peak represents the body weights of males (see Figure 7.2).

Hypothesis Testing

A well-planned investigation involves sufficient and careful thought by the investigators to define the specific question being studied. Experienced researchers routinely involve a statistician throughout the study design process to ensure that after the data have been collected, the question studied will be able to be answered in a valid and meaningful way. Statistical inference involves hypothesis testing. Statistically, it is the null hypothesis (H_0) that is tested. The H_0 states that there is no difference between treatments with respect to the outcome of interest. The research or alternative hypothesis (H_1), states that there is a difference between treatments with respect to the outcome of interest. The ability to reject or accept H_0 is dependent upon the statistical analysis of the differences observed between the groups that were studied.

Hypothesis testing is often approached in a step-wise manner:

1. Carefully define the research question to be studied and restate it in terms of the H_0 and H_1.
2. Collect data on the sample subjects.
3. Calculate the test statistic.
4. Evaluate the evidence against H_0.
5. State the conclusion.

There are two types of errors that may occur with hypothesis testing. A type I error occurs when it is falsely concluded that a significant difference exists between groups studied. It results when the null hypothesis is rejected when, in fact, it is true that no difference exists. A type II error occurs when it is falsely concluded that no significant difference exists between populations, when, in fact, a true difference exists. There are two additional terms that are important to this discussion—alpha (α) and beta (β). Alpha is defined as the probability of making a type I error; whereas, beta is defined as the probability of making a type II error. Alpha is set before data are collected, usually at 0.05. It is the

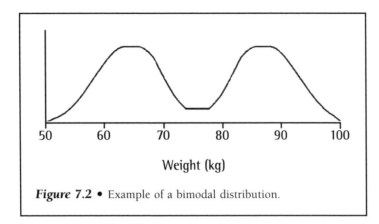

Figure 7.2 • Example of a bimodal distribution.

false-positive rate the investigators are willing to tolerate. In contrast, beta is the false-negative rate the investigators are willing to tolerate.

Statistical Power

Statistical power is the ability of a test statistic to detect a difference of a specified magnitude, if indeed a difference exists in the groups being compared. Power is the probability that a statistical test will reach a correct conclusion (i.e., declare that H_1 is true, when it really is true). When designing a study, investigators need to know how many subjects will need to complete the study in order for it to be adequately powered. In other words, the investigators need to decide upon the false negative rate they are willing to tolerate. Mathematically, power is equal to 1 – beta. Power is expressed as a percentage from 0 to 100. Most studies are powered at the 80% or 90% level. This would make beta equal to 0.2 or 0.1, respectively. When you consider that alpha is usually set at 0.05 and beta is usually set at 0.2, it is apparent that type II errors are more probable than type I errors. One of the first things a critical reader does when encountering a trial in which statistical significance was not reached (i.e., "negative trial") is to assess the power level of the study.

To determine the number of subjects needed to achieve a desired percent power, investigators must specify the following: alpha, beta, effect size, and the variability of the outcome of interest in the groups studied. Effect size is the difference that would be considered to be clinically important by practitioners. As the sample size is increased, power is increased and beta is decreased. Beta also decreases as the variability in the outcome of interest in the subjects studied decreases. As beta decreases, alpha increases. If there is a big difference between the groups being compared, power is increased and beta is decreased. This makes sense because it is much easier to see big differences than small differences. While it is generally true that the greater the power of a study the better, it is also important to realize that given a large enough sample size, anything can be statistically significant. Furthermore, simply because the results of an investigation are deemed statistically significant does not mean that they are clinically important. Conversely, just because statistical significance was not detected in an investigation does not mean that the results are not clinically important.

There are several factors that can explain why a statistical test fails to detect a significant difference of a specified effect size between groups studied. These include low power of the statistical test, small sample size, high false-negative rate for the statistical test, and, of course, the possibility that such a difference does not exist.

Sample size determination also depends on whether the test is going to be one-sided versus two-sided. A one-sided test assumes that a difference occurs in only one direction; a two-sided test looks for a difference in both the positive and negative directions. A one-sided test is more powerful than a two-sided test because regardless of the alpha chosen, a statistical test result need not vary as much from the mean value to achieve significance. For example, if alpha is set at 0.05 and the test is one-sided, the result must fall in either the top or bottom 5% of the distribution to be declared statistically significant. In contrast, if alpha is set at 0.05 and the test is two-sided, the result must fall in either the top or bottom 2.5% to be declared statistically significant.

P-values

There are several ways to explain the meaning of a p-value. A p-value is the probability of obtaining the observed difference between treatments in a study, if there is no "real" difference between treatments in the larger population of interest. It is the probability of being wrong when asserting that a true difference exists. It is also true that a p-value is the probability that the statistical observation in a study is due to chance alone. A p-value is calculated after data have been collected, and it is compared to the alpha level that was previously set to determine whether the findings are statistically significant or not.

If alpha is set at 0.05, the p-value means that if the H_0 is true, then the statistical test should discredit H_0 5% of the time or less. A p-value less than or equal to 0.05 means that the observed treatment difference is statistically different from 0. In addition, if we define a p-value less than or equal to 0.05 as being statistically significant, then we are willing to accept that 5 in 100, or 1 in 20, assertions will be wrong. It is true that, based on the alpha level that was set, the results are either deemed statistically significant or not statistically significant as determined by the calculated p-value. However, the size of the p-value does tell the reader more than just whether the results are statistically significant or not. For example, if alpha is set at 0.05 and the p-value calculated is 0.04, the results are statistically significant. Again, if alpha is set at 0.05 and the p-value calculated is 0.0001, the results are statistically significant. A p-value of 0.04 means that the probability of obtaining the observed difference between treatments in a study, if there are no "real" differences between treatments in the larger population of interest, will be about 1 in 25. Whereas a p-value of 0.0001 means that the probability of obtaining the observed difference between treatments in a study if there is no "real" difference between treatments in the larger population of interest is 1 in 10,000. Therefore, the smaller the p-value, the more certain you can be that the observed difference in the study is not merely due to chance.

A small p-value means that there is strong evidence that some difference between treatments exists—not necessarily that a large difference exists. A small p-value means that the observed differences are unlikely to be mistakes in inference due to sampling. The smaller the p-value is, the stronger the evidence against H_0.

From a literature interpretation perspective, there are a few other things to be mindful of when interpreting p-values. A p-value greater than 0.05 means that there is insufficient evidence to reject the null hypothesis H_0 at the 5% level of significance. Stating that there is insufficient evidence to demonstrate that two treatments are different does not mean that the two treatments are the same. This is a key concept. Furthermore, the size of the p-value does not indicate the clinical importance of the result. Finally, results may be statistically significant, but clinically unimportant. A limitation of p-values is that they do not tell you anything about the size or direction of the effect.

Variables and Measurement Scales

A variable is a characteristic that is being observed or measured. In a study, the dependent variable is the outcome of interest. Independent variables define the conditions under which the dependent variable is to be examined. Depending on the study, there may be no variables, one variable, or several independent variables. For example, suppose a study was planned to determine the effect of atorvastatin 20 mg daily on low-density lipoprotein (LDL) cholesterol concentrations in post-menopausal women. What is the dependent variable in this study? What is the independent variable? If you identified atorvastatin as the independent variable and LDL cholesterol concentrations as the dependent variable, you are correct. Dependent and independent variables will be discussed at greater length in the chapter on regression analysis.

Univariate and Multivariate Analysis

Depending on the number of variables being examined, researchers may conduct a univariate or multivariate analysis. Univariate analysis is used when describing one independent variable and one dependent variable. For example, investigators may be interested in estimating the annual risk of type 2 diabetes mellitus with regard to family history. In contrast, multivariate analysis is applicable to a set of observations that contain one dependent variable and more than one independent variables. For example, investigators may be interested in estimating the annual risk of type 2 diabetes mellitus with regard to family history, body mass index, ethnicity, and long-term steroid use. Statisticians use multivariate analysis to adjust for the influence of confounding variables. Multivariate analysis will be discussed in Chapters 8–10.

Types of Data

It is important to be able to identify the type of variables or data used when reading research reports, because it enables the reader to assess whether the statistical tests used were appropriate. There are two main types of data.

Continuous data are those that have constant and defined units of measurement. There is an equal distance between increments of measure. Continuous data can be further divided into interval or ratio data. The ratio scale has an absolute zero; the interval scale has the zero point arbitrarily assigned. This distinction is not important when determining the type of statistical test to use. Examples using a continuous measurement scale include blood pressure, plasma glucose concentrations, and triglyceride concentrations.

In contrast, discrete data have a limited number of categories or possible values and may be further classified as either nominal or ordinal. Nominal data are those with named or numbered categories that have no implied rank or order. The categories of a nominal scale must be exhaustive and mutually exclusive; each measurement must fall into only one category. Within any category, each individual measurement is assumed to be equivalent to the characteristic being scaled. Examples of nominal data include eye color, religious denomination, sex, presence or absence of disease, and blood type. There is no arithmetic relationship between classifications on a nominal measurement scale.

Ordinal data also have a limited number of possible categories, but they have an implied order or rank. It is important to recognize that although the order or rank is understood, the distance between each increment of measure (i.e., categories) is not equal. Examples using an ordinal measurement scale include cancer staging (e.g., stage 1, stage 2, or stage 3), New York Heart Association functional classification for patients with heart failure (class I, class II, class III, or class IV), and patient admission status (good, fair, serious, or critical).

Common Test Statistics

The type of statistical analysis and specific test statistic used depends on several factors including the type of data collected, the distribution of the data, investigator or statistician preference, the number of groups being compared, and the study design. Some common statistical tests are listed in Table 7.3. If you encounter an unfamiliar test statistic and want to learn more about it, a quick Internet search is an efficient way find additional information. Textbooks on statistics also provide detailed explanations and mathematical equations.

Statistical tests are commonly grouped into two broad categories—parametric and nonparametric. Parametric tests are generally more powerful than nonparametric tests. There are several conditions that need to be met in order to use a parametric test. The data must follow or nearly follow a normal

Table 7.3
Common Statistical Tests Used in Hypothesis Testing

	Type of Experiment				
Data type	Two Treatment Groups Consisting of Different Subjects	Three or More Treatment Groups Consisting of Different Subjects	Before and After a Single Treatment in the Same Subjects	Multiple Treatments in the Same Subjects	Associations Between Two Variables
Nominal	Chi-square or Fisher exact test if < 5 in any cell or N < 20	Chi-square or Fisher exact test if < 5 in any cell or N < 20	McNemar's test	Cochrane Q	
Ordinal	Mann-Whitney U or Wilcoxon rank sum test	Kruskal-Wallis	Wilcoxon signed rank test	Friedman statistic	
Continuous, normally distributed	t-test	Analysis of variance	Paired t-test	Repeated-measures analysis of variance	Pearson correlation
Continuous, not normally distributed	Mann-Whitney U or Wilcoxon rank sum test	Kruskal-Wallis	Wilcoxon signed rank test	Friedman statistic	Spearman rank correlation
Time-to-event	Log rank test				

Source: Reprinted with permission from Glantz SA. Primer of biostatistics. 5th ed. New York, NY: McGraw-Hill Book Co Inc; 2002.

distribution, and the variability of the data must be approximately equal between groups. Finally, the measures of patient response must be independent and unrelated, and the data must be continuous.

Nonparametric tests are used for ordinal and nominal data. In addition, if the data are continuous, but do not meet the criteria for using a parametric test, then a nonparametric test is used.

Study samples may be either independent or paired. Independent study samples are not related (i.e., the choice of subjects for one sample does not depend on which subjects are in the other sample). In contrast, paired or matched samples are related. There are a couple different ways in which study subjects can be matched: subjects may serve as their own control, such as in a cross-over trial, or subjects may be matched or paired based on specific factors that may affect the outcome of interest (e.g., age, sex, disease severity). In the latter case, one member of the matched pair is assigned to one treatment group and the other member of the matched pair is assigned to the other treatment group. The distinction between independent and matched or paired samples determines which test statistic is used.

The most commonly used parametric test is the t-test. The t-test is used to compare the means from two independent samples (i.e., two groups that have different people in each) to determine whether the null hypothesis will be accepted or rejected. When using a t-test, the null hypothesis would state that the two means of the two populations are equal. The paired t-test is used when comparing the means from a matched or paired sample (e.g., cross-over design).

If comparisons need to be made on three or more groups and the conditions for using a parametric test are met, then an analysis of variance (ANOVA) would be the preferred test. After significance has been demonstrated with ANOVA (using an F test), the researcher may want to know which groups are statistically different from each other. Post-hoc tests (also known as multiple comparison procedures) are used to compare the means of the groups two at a time to detect where the difference lies. A post-hoc test has less error associated with it than performing separate t-tests. The following are examples of post hoc tests: Bonferroni, Tukey, and Newman-Keuls.

The chi-square test is the most commonly used nonparametric test for nominal data. The chi-square test is used to check for a statistically significant association between two variables when the data are in the form of counts. This test is useful to answer research questions about rates, proportions, or frequencies on independent samples. It may also be used to answer questions about differences between proportions. Chi-square may be used if the sample size is greater than 40. However, chi-square should not be used if the sample size is less than 20. If the sample size is between 20 and 40, the expected frequency for each cell in the matrix must be greater than 5.

Fisher exact test is used instead of a chi-square if any cell in the matrix has an expected frequency of less than 5 and the sample size is between 20 and 40. This test is also preferred if the sample size is less than 20. McNemar's test is a variant of the chi-square test and is used when samples are paired. The Mantel-Haenszel chi is another variant of the chi-square test that was developed for the purpose of multivariable analysis; it is used to compare nominal data from independent samples while controlling for the effect of a confounder.

The nonparametric equivalents to the t-test for comparing two groups with independent samples when the data are ordinal include the Mann-Whitney U test and the Wilcoxon rank sum test. These tests are also appropriate when the data are continuous but not normally distributed. If the samples are paired, the appropriate test would be the Wilcoxon-signed rank test. The Kruskal-Wallis test is preferred for ordinal data when comparing three or more treatment groups with independent samples.

Survival analysis is used when investigators are interested in evaluating the time-to-the-event-of-interest for the study subjects. This statistical procedure adjusts for the fact some subjects are followed for different lengths of time. For example, in a clinical trial studying the effect of simvastatin on mortality post myocardial infarction (MI), investigators may follow each patient to one of three endpoints:

either the patient suffers another MI (event of interest), is lost to follow-up, or is alive at the conclusion of the study. Censored data refer to those from the patients who were lost to follow-up and those who are alive at the conclusion of the study. For each patient, the time between when they enrolled in the study and when they experience an endpoint is referred to the patient's survival time. The survival function, when evaluated at time (t) gives the probability that the patient will survive until at least (t). This is depicted using survival curves. A survival curve is a graph with the cumulative probability of survival on the Y-axis and the length of follow-up on the X-axis. A commonly used type of survival curve is the Kaplan-Meier. A log-rank test is used to compare relative death rates between survival curves. See Figure 7.3.

Correlation Analysis

Correlation analysis measures the strength of the association between two or more variables. Correlation analysis is used in situations where the two variables being measured change together, but neither variable can be considered to be the dependent variable. Correlation analysis measures the strength of the association between two study variables.

The correlation coefficient defines both the strength and the direction of the linear relationship between two variables. The correlation coefficient (r) can be any value from -1 to $+1$. The sign of r indicates the direction of the relationship (i.e., a positive sign indicates that as one variable increases the other variable also increases). Conversely, a negative sign indicates that as one variable increases, the other variable decreases. When r equals -1, the two variables have a perfectly negative linear relationship. In this case, all points on the scatter diagram fall exactly on a straight line that slopes downward from left to right. When r equals $+1$, the two study variables have a perfectly positive linear relationship. In this case, all points in the scatter diagram fall exactly on a straight line that slopes upward from left to right. When r equals 0, it means that there is not a linear relationship between study variables. This may mean that the relationship is either nonlinear, or it may be that the two study variables are not related.

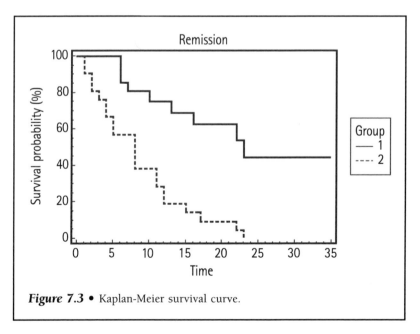

Figure 7.3 • Kaplan-Meier survival curve.

Source: MedCalc statistical software. Available at www.medcalc.be/manual/kaplan-meier.php. Accessed November 5, 2005.

The correlation coefficient, r, is a calculated statistic based on a sample that estimates the population's correlation coefficient, denoted symbolically as P. The correlation coefficient is a dimensionless value because the units in the numerator and denominator cancel. Remember that correlation does not imply causality. The existence of a statistically significant correlation between study variables does not prove that a cause-and-effect relationship exists between variables. Conversely, a statistically significant correlation between two variables does not imply that the association is clinically important. The test statistics used to determine whether the association is statistically significant or not are the Pearson correlation coefficient if the data are parametric and the Spearman rank correlation coefficient if the data are nonparametric.

Confidence Intervals

Confidence intervals provide a precise, objective way of specifying how good a sample estimate is, taking into account both sample size and variability. Because the value of the computed sample statistic varies from sample to sample, uncertainty enters the estimation process. A confidence interval defines boundaries within which the true population parameter is likely to fall. Various confidence levels are encountered in the health sciences literature; however, the most common is the 95% confidence interval. It is computed as follows: 95% CI = $(\overline{X}) \pm 1.96$ (SEM).

Since all of the possible values of the sample mean tend to follow a normal distribution, the true, but unmeasured, mean in the larger population of interest will lie within two standard errors of the sample mean about 95% of the time. This means that if you repeated an experiment 100 times and generated a confidence interval for each time you repeated the experiment, then 95 of the confidence intervals will contain the true, but unmeasured, mean in the larger population of interest and 5 of the confidence intervals will not. Confidence intervals are the range of possible values for the true treatment difference that are statistically likely given the results of a specific trial. Confidence intervals are most commonly used to estimate the true, but unmeasured, mean value in the larger population of interest for continuous data that are normally distributed, but may also be calculated for medians, regression slopes, relative risks, hazard ratios, etc.

Referring back to the example of measuring SBPs in 100 first-year pharmacy students, the calculated SEM equals 1 mmHg. It would be correct to state that you may be 95% confident that the true, but unmeasured, mean SBP in all first-year pharmacy students will be contained in the range of 108 mmHg to 112 mmHg, inclusive. It would be incorrect to state that 95 of the 100 first-year pharmacy students in the sample had SBPs in the range of 108 mmHg to 112 mmHg. SD is used to describe the subject-to-subject variability with a data set, and SEM is used to describe the sample-to-sample variation among all possible values of the sample mean. This is an important distinction.

Confidence intervals convey more information to readers than p-values. Confidence intervals provide information regarding the size and direction of effect observed. When interpreting confidence intervals, any value from the lower confidence bound up to and including the upper confidence bound could be the true value in the larger population of interest. Confidence intervals also allow the reader to determine whether a finding is statistically significant or not simply by looking at the interval. The first step in doing this is to determine whether you are looking at a ratio (e.g., hazard ratio, risk ratio, odds ratio) or anything else (e.g., mean, standard deviation). If you are in the "anything else" category, and the confidence interval includes 0, then you may conclude that statistical significance is not achieved. This is because statistically it is the H_0 (i.e., the hypothesis of no difference that is being tested). Therefore, if the confidence interval crosses 0, the possibility of no difference between groups exists, and it is correct to conclude that statistical significance has not been achieved. Conversely, if the confidence interval does not include 0, it is correct to conclude that statistical significance has been achieved.

If you are evaluating a confidence interval for a ratio, the same logic applies, but now the magic number for determining whether or not a finding is statistically significant is 1. Therefore, if the confidence interval crosses 1, the possibility of no difference between groups exists, and it is correct to conclude that statistical significance has not been achieved. Conversely, if the confidence interval does not include 1, it is correct to conclude that statistical significance has been achieved. Remember, that statistically it is the H_0 that is being tested. Visually, a ratio is represented as A/B, if A equals 2 and B equals 2, then the ratio would be expressed as 2/2, and 2/2 is 1; hence, the magic number to determine whether statistical significance is achieved when looking at a confidence interval for a ratio is 1.

The width of a confidence interval can be affected by several factors. Given a fixed standard deviation, increasing the number of people in the sample will narrow the width of a confidence interval. Decreasing the confidence level will also narrow the width of a confidence interval (e.g., going from 95% CI to an 80% CI). In addition, the lower the individual variation among persons in the population from which the sample is drawn, the narrower the confidence interval.

Although the confidence interval method is useful and provides the reader with more information compared with a p-value, it cannot control for errors in study design or improper selection of study subjects.

Calculating Measures of Association

Calculating relative risk, relative risk reduction, absolute risk reduction, and numbers needed to treat can be helpful when trying to determine the clinical applicability of results published in a research report. Organizing the results of a trial into a 2-by-2 table (Table 7.4) and using the equations provided below enables the reader to compute these measures of association.[4]

Relative risk (RR) compares the probability of an outcome among individuals who have a specified characteristic or who have been exposed to a risk factor to the probability of that outcome among individuals who lack the characteristic or who have not been exposed to a risk factor. In the context of a clinical trial evaluating drug A compared with placebo, it is the ratio of risk of an event occurring in the group that received drug A compared to the risk of the event occurring in the group that received placebo. Interpretation of RR focuses on the number 1. A RR less than 1 indicates that the therapy decreased the risk of developing the adverse outcome in the group that received drug A compared with the group that received placebo. An RR equal to 1 means that there is no difference in outcomes between treatment with drug A and placebo. An RR greater than 1 means that treatment with drug A increased the risk of developing the adverse outcome compared with placebo. It is important to note that relative risk is only applicable to prospective cohort trials. This is because, by definition, RR requires that it is known in advance whether the patients will receive active treatment or control. The following equation is used to calculate relative risk.[4]

$$RR = [A / (A + B)]/[C / (C + D)]$$

Table 7.4
Exposure and Outcome

	Primary Outcome Yes	Primary Outcome No	Total
Exposure	A	B	A + B
No Exposure	C	D	C + D

Table 7.5
Simvastatin and Placebo

	Nonfatal MI or Death from CHD Yes	Nonfatal MI or Death from CHD No	Total
Simvastatin 40 mg, daily	144	4151	4295
Placebo, daily	296	3704	4000

Absolute risk reduction (ARR) is defined as the difference in the risk of the outcome between subjects who have received treatment and those who have received another. This measure provides the percentage of patients spared the adverse outcome as the result of receiving the experimental rather than the control therapy. Absolute risk reduction changes with a change in baseline risk. An ARR of 0 indicates no difference between comparison groups. The following equation is used to calculate an absolute risk reduction.[4]

$$ARR = [C / (C + D)] - [A / (A + B)]$$

Relative risk reduction (RRR) estimates the percentage of baseline risk that is removed as a result of therapy. This is the percent reduction in the experimental group event rate compared with the control group event rate. This measure is used to compare the efficacy of treatment to that of the control group. If the RRR is equal to 0, then there was no effect of the treatment compared with the control in terms of the outcome of interest. Mathematically, relative risk reduction is 1 − RR multiplied by 100. The following equation may also be used to calculate relative risk reduction.[4]

$$RRR = \{[C / (C + D) - [A / (A + B)]\} / [C / (C + D)]$$

The number needed to treat (NNT) indicates the number of patients who require treatment to prevent one event, and it can help us use data to make better clinical decisions. Keep in mind that NNT assumes that baseline risk is the same for all patients in the larger population of interest. The following equation is used to calculate numbers needed to treat.[4]

$$NNT = 1 / ARR$$
$$NNT = 1/ [C / (C + D)] - [A / (A + B)]$$

Use the following information to practice computing RR, RRR, ARR, and NNT. A trial was conducted to determine the efficacy of simvastatin in preventing coronary events in women with moderate hypercholesterolemia and no history of myocardial infarction (MI). A total of 8295 patients were randomized to either simvastatin 40 mg, given orally, daily (n = 4295) or matching placebo (n = 4000). The average length of patient follow-up was 6.2 years. The primary endpoint was the occurrence of nonfatal MI or death from coronary heart disease (CHD). These two endpoints were combined. One hundred forty-four patients treated with simvastatin and 296 patients treated with placebo experienced the combined endpoint. The first step is to set up the 2-by-2 table correctly (Table 7.5). Then using the equations above, compute each measure of association. If you computed RR to be 0.445; ARR to be 4.1%; RRR =to be 55%, and NNT to be 24 patients, you are correct.

Acknowledgement: The author gratefully acknowledges Mr. Brian Cole for his illustrations.

References

1. Knopp RH, Gitter H, Truitt T, Bays H, Manion CV, Lipka LJ, et al. Effects of ezetimibe, a new cholesterol absorption inhibitor, on plasma lipids in patients with primary hypercholesterolemia. *Eur Heart J.* 2003;24(8):729–741.
2. Heymsfield SB, Segal KR, Hauptman J, Lucas CP, Boldrin MN, Rissanen A, et al. Effects of weight loss with orlistat on glucose tolerance and pro-gression to type 2 diabetes in obese adults. *Arch Intern Med.* 2000;160(9):1321–1326.
3. Glantz SA. *Primer of Biostatistics.* 5th ed. New York: McGraw-Hill; 2002.
4. Kendrach MG, Covington TR, McCarthy MW, Harris MC. Calculating risks and number-needed-to-treat: method of data interpretation. *J Manage Care Pharm.*1997;3:179–183.

Additional Reading

Ascione FJ. *Principles of Scientific Literature Evaluation: Critiquing Clinical Drug Trials.* Washington DC: American Pharmaceutical Association; 2001.

Friedman LM, Furberg CD, DeMets DL. *Fundamentals of Clinical Trials.* 3rd ed. New York: Springer; 1998.

Gaddis ML, Gaddis GM. Introduction to biostatistics: part 1, basic concepts. *Ann Emerg Med.* 1990;19:86–89.

Gaddis ML, Gaddis GM. Introduction to biostatistics: part 2, descriptive statistics. *Ann Emerg Med.* 1990;19:309–315.

Gaddis ML, Gaddis GM. Introduction to biostatistics: part 3, sensitivity, specificity, predictive value, and hypothesis testing. *Ann Emerg Med.* 1990;19:820–825.

Gaddis ML, Gaddis GM. Introduction to biostatistics: part 4, statistical inference techniques in hypothesis testing. *Ann Emerg Med.* 1990;19:820–825.

Gaddis ML, Gaddis GM. Introduction to biostatistics: part 5, statistical inference techniques in hypothesis testing with nonparametric data. *Ann Emerg Med.* 1990;19:1054–1059.

Gaddis ML, Gaddis GM. Introduction to biostatistics: part 6, correlation and regression. *Ann Emerg Med.* 1990;19:1462–1468.

Garb JL. *Understanding Medical Research: A Practitioner's Guide.* Boston: Little, Brown and Company; 1996.

Gehlbach SH. *Interpreting the Medical Literature.* 4th ed. New York: McGraw-Hill; 2002.

Goldman L, Ausiello D, eds. *Cecil Textbook of Medicine.* 22nd ed. Philadelphia: W.B. Saunders; 2004.

Hirsch RP, Riegelman RK. *Statistical First Aid: Interpretation of Health Research Data.* Boston: Blackwell Scientific Publications; 1992.

Knapp RG, Miller MC. *Clinical Epidemiology and Biostatistics.* Baltimore, MD: Williams & Wilkins; 1992.

Last A, Wilson S. Relative risk and odds ratio: what's the difference? *J Fam Pract.* 2004;53(2). Available online at: www.jfponline.com/content/2004/02/jfp_0204_00108.asp. Accessed March 1, 2005.

Riegelman RK, Hirsch RP. *Studying a Study and Testing a Test: How to Read the Health Science Literature.* 3rd ed. Boston: Little, Brown and Company; 1996.

Sackett DL, Haynes RB, Guyatt GH, Tugwell P. *Clinical Epidemiology: Aa Basic Science for Clinical Medicine.* 2nd ed. Boston: Little, Brown and Company; 1991.

Spilker B. *Guide to Clinical Trials.* Philadelphia: Lippincott, Williams & Wilkins; 1991.

Stolley PD, Strom BL. Sample size calculations for clinical pharmacology studies. *Clin Pharmacol Ther.* 1986;39(5):489–490.

Section Three

Regression Analysis

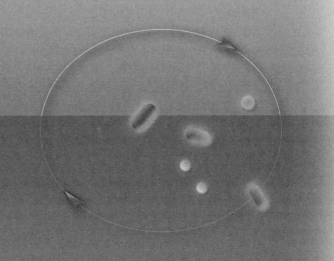

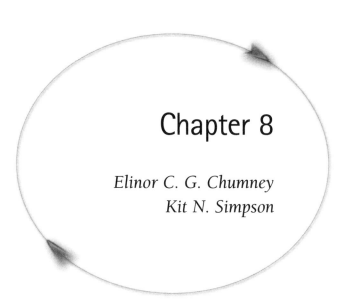

Chapter 8

Elinor C. G. Chumney
Kit N. Simpson

Introduction to Regression Analysis

Many variables are interactive or predictive of one another, and there are a wide variety of analytic tools that researchers can use to untangle and define these relationships. We will briefly introduce a number of these tools here, mainly correlation and various regression techniques. The key for any researcher is to first choose the correct analytic tool to address the question at hand and then to focus on correctly interpreting the results.

Pearson Correlation

Often, a research question can be reduced to the relationship between two continuous random variables, such as total cholesterol levels and patient age. In this case, a Pearson correlation coefficient (r) can be used to provide a measure of both how strongly and in what direction these two variables are linearly related.

The strength of the linear relationship between the two variables is reflected in the absolute value or magnitude of the correlation coefficient. If $|r| = 1$ then all of the observations in the sample, i.e., on a straight line when plotted on a two-dimensional axis; a perfect linear relationship. If there is no linear relationship at all between the two variables, then $r = 0$. The stronger the relationship, the closer the absolute value of r is to 1. For example, $|r|=.67$ indicates a much stronger linear relationship than $|r|=.15$.

A positive sign on the correlation coefficient indicates a positive relationship between the two variables, such that as one increases the other also tends to increase.

Because we generally expect total cholesterol levels to increase as a patient ages, we would expect a positive correlation coefficient between these two variables.

Similarly, a negative sign on the correlation coefficient indicates a negative relationship between the two variables, such that as one increases the other tends to decrease. For example, we generally expect bone density levels to decrease as a patient ages, so we would expect a negative correlation coefficient between these two variables.

There are three main drawbacks to using correlation coefficients. The first is that a researcher is limited to testing for a linear relationship. The second is that a simple correlation does not control for other relevant information (such as gender, prescription drug use, weight, and exercise levels in the examples discussed above). And finally, correlation does not imply causation. The fact that two variables are correlated does not necessarily mean that one caused the other.

Linear Regression

Although correlation is not concerned with causation, a related statistical procedure is. The correlations we observed above for both total cholesterol levels and bone density measures are essentially simple linear regressions; also known as ordinary least squares (OLS) regression. This technique is used to forecast or predict the value of a dependent variable (Y) based on the value of a single explanatory variable (X), using the following formula:

$$Y = \beta_0 + \beta_1 X_1 + e$$

Recall that this is the algebraic formula for a straight line. The data is plotted on a two-dimensional axis with Y values on the vertical axis and X values on the horizontal axis. The stronger the correlation between the two variables, then more the data points will appear to lie on a straight line. The β_0 indicates the intercept, where the plotted line intercepts the Y axis, and the β_1 indicates the slope, the amount of change in Y associated with a one-unit change in X.

Because only rarely will all of the points fall exactly on a straight line (as they would in the case of perfect correlation), the error term e is included in the equation notation. To judge the goodness of fit of a regression (i.e., how closely the points converge on the estimated line), researchers examine the R-squared value. In a simple linear regression with only one explanatory variable, this is simply the square of the correlation coefficient (r).

A special type of simple linear regression is commonly known as a one-way ANOVA (analysis of variance). The analysis assesses the effect of a categorical explanatory variable on Y by testing for different mean values of Y across the various categories of X.

But rarely is there just one expected cause for a given dependent variable. Unlike a simple linear regression or correlation, a multiple linear regression analysis allows researchers to examine more than one relationship at a time. In doing so, they can (1) isolate the effect of one explanatory variable (X) on Y from the other X's (i.e., controlling for the other X's) and (2) forecast or predict the value of Y based on the value of a series of explanatory variables. The coefficients of a multiple regression equation give the change in response per unit change in a predictor when all other predictors are held fixed.

OLS regression, analyzing the relationship between a continuous dependent variable and potentially a number of independent variables, is discussed in greater detail in Chapter 9. However, it is limited to examining linear associations and does not perform well in nonlinear cases.

Logistic Regression

In many cases, the dependent variable of interest is categorical, such as the success or failure of a particular drug therapy. When this is the case, logistic and not OLS regression is appropriate. The regression formula may be structured similarly, but in this case the dependent variable (Y) is the probability of some event, such as the success of a particular drug therapy.

$$Y = (\text{Probability of success}) = \beta_0 + \beta_1 X_1 + e$$

Researchers can compute odds ratios (OR) for each explanatory variable (X) based on the individual parameter estimates, and they can use the full logistic equation to predict the probability of a particular outcome of interest. This method of analysis is discussed in greater detail in Chapter 10.

Sample Selection Models

Finally, there are cases where the dependent variable of interest is censored in some way. When this happens, the subset of data we observe is not representative of the population as a whole. Sample selection bias refers to problems where the dependent variable is only observed for a restricted, nonrandom sample. Sample selection bias is quite common in studies that assess the outcomes for patients using data from observational patient cohorts or other "real practice" settings. We may observe sample selection bias that is due to "confounding by indication." This is the case when a new treatment or drug is used more often for patients who are sicker, more difficult to treat because they have comorbid conditions, or because they receive treatment in a setting, such as an academic medical center, where new therapies are adopted more rapidly than in other less "technology friendly" settings. Researchers often try to control for differences in disease severity or the presence of comorbid conditions through the use of severity or risk adjustment measures. However, limitations in the type of clinical variables that can control for disease severity, the risk of hospital admission, or the presence of comorbidities may in turn limit the researchers' ability to control statistically for population differences. Furthermore, we can never be certain that these types of control variable truly remove the total effect of any selection bias.

In recent years it has become common practice to use one of a number of approaches to examine the results for effects due to selection bias. Researchers can use an instrumental variable (IV) approach, a propensity score approach, or a two stage Heckman modeling approach. These methods are computationally complex, but conceptually easy to understand. They attempt to compensate statistically for the fact that either (1) the observational data on the treatments of interest have been derived from populations that do not have the same likelihood of benefiting due to "confounding by indication," or (2) that the observed outcomes or costs are for groups of patients who do not have the same propensity (likelihood) of being hospitalized, likelihood of having costly comorbid conditions, or risk of having high number of cases with very severe disease. In-depth explanations of these approaches can be found in papers by Rubin (1997), McClellan (1994), and Wexler (2004).[1-3]

The use of these methods for examining regression models for sample selection bias is relatively new in outcomes research, and many fairly recently published studies do not employ them. This is unfortunate, because sample selection bias may affect any observational cohort of patients. We have no way of knowing if the outcomes reported for patient groups in noncontrolled studies may actually be attributed to selection bias if the authors have not attempted to examine this issue by using one of the sample selection bias control methods described here. Increasing pressure from peer reviewers and journal editors should make it increasingly difficult to get an observational study published if the authors have not used one of these methods to test their findings for sample selection bias. Please see the appendix for a more in-depth treatment of this subject.

Introduction of Data

Throughout the next three chapters, we will present data from an antiretroviral trial in patients who had not previously received any highly active antiretroviral therapy (HAART). Patients were randomized to a new HAART regimen (a combination of three drugs, one a new protease inhibitor) compared to the most powerful HAART regimen currently on the market. At the conclusion of the trial, researchers will want to know whether the new drug treatment has had a positive effect on patient outcomes, as measured by a decrease in viral load (VL) levels.

For the linear regression analysis, the dependent variable (Y) will be a measure of the patient's VL transformed to the logarithmic scale. This transformation is usual in clinical trials involving measures of VL, and a clinically significant improvement over baseline VL levels would be about a 0.5 log decrease.

This linear regression analysis will allow researchers to measure the expected decrease in patient VL levels. However, because a primary goal of treatment for HIV is to reduce VL levels to the point that they are no longer detectable, they may also want to undertake a logistic regression analysis to assess how well they are meeting that treatment goal. As just discussed, the dependent variable (Y) is dichotomous in a logistic regression. Whether the VL is detectable is predicted using the same explanatory variables described above. Clearly, an undetectable VL is the most desirable treatment outcome in recent clinical trials of new HIV-disease therapies.

To assess whether the new drug caused a significant drop in VL levels, the researchers will include it as the primary explanatory variable in both the linear and logistic regression analyses. They will measure it as a dichotomous variable with a value of 1 if the patient received the new drug and a value of 0 if the patient did not.

A number of other explanatory variables which could conceivably influence patient outcomes will also be included in the model. These include a patient's baseline VL level, age, and whether or not he or she uses intravenous (IV) drugs. A measure of a patient's VL levels at the beginning of the study will be included to control for severity. Sicker patients may respond less well to a given treatment, or the opposite could be the case. Because some studies have indicated that IV drug users may respond less well to HIV drug therapy, a dichotomous variable will also be included to indicate whether or not the patient was an IV drug user.

Patient age was measured as a continuous variable, but the researchers will transform it into a series of dichotomous variables. For the Age 30–44 variable, patients will be coded with a value of either 1 (if they fall in that age range) or 0 (if they are either older or younger). Similarly, for the Age 45+ variable, patients will be coded with a value of either 1 (if they fall in that age range) or 0 (if they are younger). The researchers will compare the experience of these two age groups to the reference age category of <30. Patients who are less than 30 will be identified as those coded with a 0 for the other two age categories. Accordingly, the reference age category does not appear as a unique variable in the equations; it is the omitted variable.

Finally, the researchers may decide to include an interaction term to assess whether the new drug works significantly differently for patients with either very high or very low baseline viral loads. A description of all variables that will be discussed in the following chapters is included in Table 8.1. Please refer to it as you read the model descriptions in Chapters 9 and 10.

Conclusion

There are many factors to consider when deciding which model is most appropriate for the research question at hand. OLS works well with continuous dependent variables, and logistic regression is appropriate for categorical dependent variables. These two approaches will be discussed in greater detail in the following chapters, and the examples therein will be based on the data just introduced.

Table 8.1
Variables Used to Model a Patient's Drop in Viral Load with New Drug Therapy

Variable Type	Variable Name	Description
Treatment Variable	New Drug	Dichotomous variable indicating whether or not the patient received the new drug
Patient characteristics	Baseline Viral Load (Log Base 10)	Log-transformed measure of the patient's viral load at the beginning of the study
	IV Drug User	Dichotomous variable indicating whether or not the patient is an IV drug user
	Age categories	
	Age < 30	Reference (i.e., omitted) age category
	Age 30–44	Dichotomous variable indicating whether or not the patient is between the ages of 30 and 44
	Age 45+	Dichotomous variable indicating whether or not the patient is age 45 or older
Interaction term	New Drug Baseline Viral Load	Product of the New Drug and Baseline Viral Load variables already included in the model

References

1. McClellan M, McNeil BJ, Newhouse JP. Does more intensive treatment of acute myocardial infarction in the elderly reduce mortality? *JAMA*. 1994;272:859–866.

2. Rubin DB. Estimating causal effects from large data sets using propensity scores. *Ann Int Med*. 1997;127(S8):757–763.

3. Wexler DJ, Chen J, Smith GL, Radford MJ, Yaari S, Bradford WD, Krumholz HM. Predictors of costs of caring for elderly patients discharged with heart failure. *Am Heart J*. 2001;142(2):350–357.

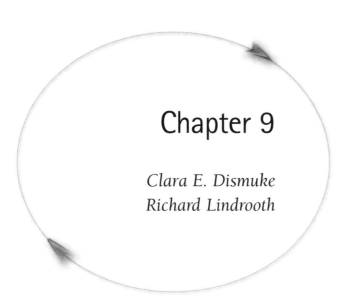

Chapter 9

Clara E. Dismuke
Richard Lindrooth

Ordinary Least Squares

Ordinary least squares, referred to as OLS, is one of the most common techniques used in multivariate analysis. Regrettably, it is also probably the technique most misused. In this chapter, we describe the assumptions behind OLS estimation and the situations where it is most valid. We conclude with a short description of extensions to OLS that are designed to overcome its shortcomings in specific situations.

Ordinary Least Squares Defined

The method of OLS has been understood for close to 200 years. The remarkable innovation behind OLS is the recognition that there could be errors in the relationship between dependent and explanatory variables. Consider the following simple identity:

$$\text{Area of a Circle} = \pi \, (\text{Radius}^2)$$

There is no error in an identity; it is always true. Thus, π is easily solved for with data on the area of the circle and the radius:

$$\pi = \text{Area of a Circle}/(\text{Radius}^2)$$

Of course, the value of π is well known, but if one only had information on the area of a circle and the radius (and was ignorant of π), he or she could solve for the precise value of π with complete certainty assuming that there was no error in measurement.

OLS is useful when the parameters are unknown and the relationship between the dependent variable and the explanatory variable is a hypothesis that needs to be tested. For example, consider the relationship between a measured drop in viral load of HIV positive patients and the baseline viral load:

$$\text{Drop Viral Load} = \beta_0 + \beta_1 \, \text{Baseline Viral Load}$$

Here, β_0 and β_1 are unknown parameters. This relationship can be graphed, where β_0 represents an intercept term and β_1 is a slope coefficient. Figure 9-1 graphs individual observations of the drop in viral load and the baseline viral load and the line represented by OLS estimation of β_0 and β_1. Note that each observation is off the line; thus, baseline viral load is not a perfect predictor of the subsequent drop. The appropriate model is really:

$$\text{DropVL} = \beta_0 + \beta_1 \, \text{BaseVL} + \varepsilon,$$

where ε is the random error in the model, dropVL is the log drop in viral load, and baseVL is the baseline viral load. Graphically, the vertical difference between the line and the observation (i.e., the dotted lines) is called the residual. The line is derived using OLS and can be estimated using virtually any statistical or spreadsheet software package. As before, the parameter β_0 is the intercept term and β_1 is the slope of the line.

The values for the parameters β_0 and β_1 minimize the sum of the squared vertical distance between the points and the line, or the sum of squared residuals:

$$\sum_{i=1}^{N} \varepsilon_i^2$$

where N is the number of observations in the sample. The "least squares" part of ordinary least squares reflects the fact that the OLS estimate of the parameters is the one that yields the least (or minimum) sum of squared residuals. In summary, OLS is implemented as follows:

1. Calculate the distance between each observation and a line
   - The distance between the fitted line and the observation is the residual

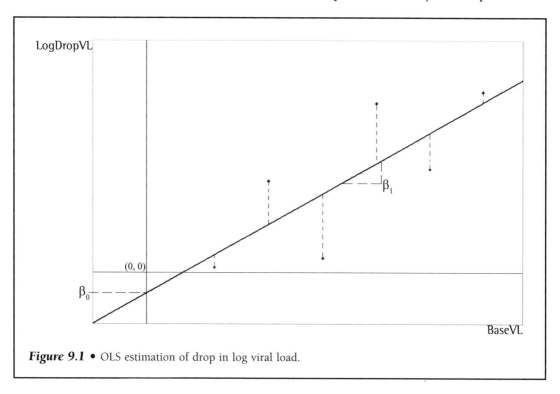

Figure 9.1 • OLS estimation of drop in log viral load.

- When the observation lies on the line, then the residual is 0
- The better the line fits the data, the smaller the residuals will be
2. Square the residual so that the positive and negative residuals (i.e., where the points lie above or below the fitted line, respectively) don't cancel each other out
3. Pick the line that minimizes the sum of the squared residuals

This method of minimizing the sum of squared residuals is numerically equivalent to the method of maximum likelihood, which will be discussed in more detail later in the book. Maximum likelihood estimates yield parameters such that the likelihood of being able to use those parameters (and the model) to replicate the actual data is maximized. Because OLS is linear, this is equivalent to minimizing the sum of squared errors. Note, however, that both OLS and maximum likelihood take the structure of the model (e.g., linearity) as given and only find the parameters that satisfy the objective function. Thus, if the underlying model is wrong, neither OLS nor maximum will yield the true estimates.

Interpreting Coefficients

A dependent variable is usually denoted Y in a regression model and is presented on the left-hand side. The independent variables are usually denoted as a series of Xs. We adopt this custom when we are speaking generally about the OLS method. In our example, the dependent variable is *dropVL*. It is easy to remember which is the dependent variable because it is the variable whose value is *dependent* on the values of the other independent variables in the model. All other variables are independent variables.

Since we want to analyze the effect of the new drug on the decrease in viral load, we will enter a binary (equal to 0 if the patient did not get the drug and 1 if he or she did) variable to measure the effect of the drug:

$$DropVL = \beta_0 + \beta_1 \text{ New Drug} + \beta_2 \text{ BaseVL} + \varepsilon$$

Figure 9.2 displays the effect of including a binary variable in the regression. Note that binary variables are often called *dummy variables*. When the binary variable equals 0, indicating no drug treatment, the relationship between the baseline viral load and the drop in viral load is represented by the bottom line in the graph. When the binary variable equals 1, indicating treatment with the new drug, the relationship is represented by the top line in the graph. The vertical distance between the two lines reflects the effectiveness of the new drug. Thus, according to this simple model, the new drug leads to an equal drop in the viral load no matter what the baseline viral load.

However, it may be that the new drug is more effective on people with a higher baseline viral load than on those with low baseline viral loads. In other words, the magnitude of the drop might increase as the baseline viral load increases. We can model this possibility by including an interaction term. An interaction term is two variables multiplied by one another. Thus, the new specification is:

$$DropVL = \beta_0 + \beta_1 \text{ New Drug} + \beta_2 \text{ BaseVL} + \beta_3 \text{ New Drug} \times \text{BaseVL} + \varepsilon$$

Here, β_1 reflects the effect of the new drug, regardless of the baseline viral load and β_3 measures the effect of the new drug on the slope of the line. Thus, a positive β_3 can be interpreted to mean that the effect of the new drug on the drop in viral load is greater as the baseline viral load increases. Figure 9.3 displays the effect of including a binary variable and an interaction term in the regression. When new drug = 0 (indicating no drug treatment), the relationship between drop in viral load and baseline viral

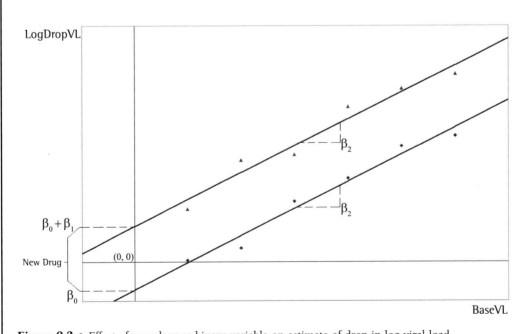

Figure 9.2 • Effect of new drug as binary variable on estimate of drop in log viral load.

load is represented by the lower line. In contrast, when new drug = 1 (indicating drug treatment), the relationship is reflected by the top line. Note that, as in Figure 9.2, the drop in viral load is greater for all patients with the new drug. However, the lines are no longer parallel, due to the interaction term. When we include the interaction, we can observe that the effect of the new drug is greater as the baseline viral load increases.

Goodness of Fit and Hypothesis Tests

The R-squared statistic, denoted R^2, measures the "goodness of fit" of a regression line. It is the proportion of the variance of the dependent variable that can be explained by the independent variables. The value of R^2 ranges between 0 and 1. If R^2 is close to 1, then the relationship between the dependent and independent variables is precise. Recall that in Figure 9.1 there was quite a bit of space between the individual data points and the regression line. The R^2 for this regression in Figure 9.1 is likely to be in the 0.2–0.4 range. If the individual data points were instead very close to the line, then the R^2 would be closer to 1. Consider the identity:

$$\text{Area of a Circle} = \pi \, (\text{Radius}^2)$$

A regression of the area of the circle on radius squared would yield an R^2 of exactly 1 because the radius squared will explain all of the variation in the area of a circle.

We usually consider $R^2 > 0.30$ (meaning the model explains 30% of the variation in Y) to be quite good in cross-sectional analyses. However, a drawback of R^2 is that it always increases as additional variables are added to an equation, even if they are completely irrelevant. Thus, focusing solely on maximizing R^2 is a bad idea.

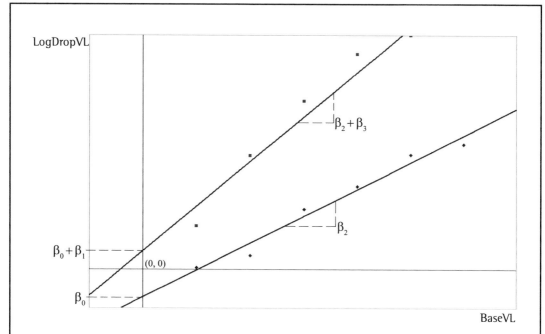

Figure 9.3 • Effect of adding interaction term between new drug and baseline viral load.

Adjusted R^2 is another measure of the "goodness of fit" of a regression line. Adjusted R^2 has been adjusted for the number of independent variables in the model. It can vary outside of the 0–1 range. It can either increase or decrease as additional variables are added to an equation, depending on whether the additional variables are substantively important in the model. The adjusted R^2 will be lower as extraneous variables are added to the model.

Hypothesis tests can be performed to assess whether the parameter estimates are statistically significant. The null hypothesis is usually that the parameter estimate is equal to 0, meaning that the variable X has no effect on the dependent variable Y. The alternative hypothesis is that the parameter estimate is different than 0; the variable X does indeed have a discernible effect on Y. Thus, the standard test is two-sided. The test statistic is the estimated parameter divided by its standard error. Standard errors are calculated using the sum of squared residuals and the standard deviation of the X variables. The larger the variation in the residuals (i.e., the farther from the OLS line each observation falls), the larger the standard error.

The test statistic for a single parameter is evaluated using either a t-distribution or a normal distribution. P-values are calculated based on the distribution. A small p-value indicates more confidence that a particular variable X contributes significantly to explaining the observed variance in the dependent variable Y. Usually the t-distribution is used if the number of observations is small. As the number of observations increases, the t-distribution begins to look like a normal distribution. Accordingly, the normal distribution is used when the number of observations is quite large (after 30 degrees of freedom).

A p-value = 0.05 indicates that the researcher should be 95% confident that the parameter estimate is statistically significant. Similarly, a p-value of 0.01 implies 99% confidence that the parameter is different from 0. In other words, an observed p-value less than 0.05 would imply we should reject the null hypothesis that the parameter is 0. Conversely, when an observed p-value is high (i.e., above 0.05), then the researcher is unable to reject the null that the parameters are 0. The statistical standard of at least 95% confidence (i.e., p-value < 0.05) is very high. However, in some applications, it is acceptable to treat a p-value of less than 0.10 as significant, especially if the parameter is considered to be clinically significant.

Related to these tests is the concept of confidence intervals (C.I.). Researchers sometimes report 95% confidence intervals, which shows the range of the parameter estimates within which the researcher is 95% confident the true parameter lies. If the confidence interval does not include 0, then the parameter is statistically significant.

Numerical Example

There are several assumptions that are necessary for the validity of the OLS estimates. However, before we proceed to the assumptions, we will give an example using real data. Our data is from an actual clinical trial to evaluate the effect of a new drug designed to reduce the viral load in individuals with HIV disease. In order to accomplish this, we will use ordinary least squares to estimate a model where the dependent variable (Y) is the decrease in viral load measured in log base 10. We know *a priori* that a 0.5 drop in log viral load is clinically significant.

In earlier examples, we did not include any other variables that might explain the drop in the viral load, such as, patient characteristics. In this example, we will also control for the influence of other important patient characteristics on viral load, including whether or not the individual is an intravenous drug user, entered as a binary (equal to 0 if no, 1 if yes) variable, and age categories.

Sometimes age is entered as a continuous variable, but we choose to enter it as a series of categorical variables since older HIV patients may experience different outcomes with the drug than younger patients, and this effect is easier to observe with age expressed in categories. So, we created three binary age variables (equal to 0 if the patient is not in that age group and equal to 1 if the patient is in that age group): one for individuals younger than 30, one for individuals between the ages of 30 and 44, and one for individuals age 45 and older. It is always necessary to omit one of the categorical or dummy variables in estimating an OLS model in order to avoid perfect multicollinearity which would occur if all categories are included. We omit the younger than 30 category in the specification below.

Our final specification is thus:

$$\text{DropVL} = \beta_0 + \beta_1 \text{ NewDrug} + \beta_2 \text{ BaseVL} + \beta_3 \text{ NewDrug} \times \text{BaseVL} + \beta_4 \text{ IVDU} + \beta_5 \text{ Age30–44} + \beta_6 \text{ Age45} + \varepsilon$$

In this model, β_0 represents the constant term, β_1 the coefficient on the new drug, β_2 the coefficient on base viral load, β_3 the coefficient on the interaction, β_4 the coefficient on intravenous drug use, β_5 the coefficient on age 30 to 44, and β_6 the coefficient on age 45 and older. The coefficients on the continuous variable will indicate the magnitude of change in the dependent variable with a one-unit change in that continuous (nonbinary) variables. In this case, only baseline viral load is entered as a continuous variable, and its coefficient. The coefficients on the binary variables show the change in the dependent variable when the binary variable changes from 0 to 1. All coefficients represent partial effects and are interpreted as the change in the dependent variable, $\log_{10}$ drop in viral load, when that particular factor is changed, holding all the other variables constant.

We present in Table 9.1 the model estimated with and without an interaction term. Implicit in the equation above is the assumption that the differential effect of the *new drug* binary variable is constant across all levels of the baseline viral load and that the differential effect of baseline viral load is also constant regardless of whether or not the patient is in the new drug group. If for some reason the effects of taking or not taking the new drug on viral load drop varies by the baseline viral load, then a new variable which is an interaction (multiplication) of these two variables should be included in the model.

We estimate the model using Huber-White (robust) standard errors to correct for the potential problem of heteroscedasticity (see the Violations section). In the presence of heteroscedasticity, the standard errors will usually be too small and the t-statistics are biased upward.

In addition to the coefficient estimates on each variable, we show the standard errors of the estimates in parentheses and the p-values in brackets. We also show the number of observations (patients in this case) and the R^2, which represents the amount of variance in the dependent variable ($\log_{10}$ of the viral load drop) described by the model.

Recall that the C.I. is a range of values around our parameter estimate. This range reflects alternative values that are not significantly different than our point estimate. We define statistical significance as a 0.05 p-value or 95% confidence. For example, if 0 fell within our confidence interval, then we would *fail* to reject a hypothesis that our estimate is statistically significant from 0. The results from this first equation (without the interaction term) indicate that maintaining all other factors constant, when patients are put on the new drug therapy, the expected drop in their $\log_{10}$ viral load is 0.747 (C.I. 0.727–0.768). According to the literature, since this is above 0.5, the drop is clinically significant.

We can similarly analyze the effect of the other factor that is significant, baseline viral load. We estimate that with a one-unit increase in baseline viral load, the drop in $\log_{10}$ viral load is 0.838 (C.I. 0.818–0.859). Though we include age and intravenous drug use in our model based on a theoretical

Table 9.1
Ordinary Least Squares Estimates

Variables	Model Without Interaction	Model With Interaction
Constant	-0.451**	-0.116
	(0.054)	(0.079)
	[0.000]	[0.142]
New drug	0.747**	0.014
	(0.010)	(0.079)
	[0.000]	[0.860]
Baseline viral load (log base 10)	0.838**	0.772**
	(0.010)	(0.014)
	[0.000]	[0.000]
IV drug user	0.002	0.001
	(0.019)	(0.014)
	[0.904]	[0.930]
Age 30–44	0.001	-0.005
	(0.014)	(0.011)
	[0.920]	[0.660]
Age 45+	0.030	0.025*
	(0.016)	(0.011)
	[0.054]	[0.024]
New drug* baseline viral load		0.147**
		(0.015)
		[0.000]
Number of observations	232	232
R-squared	0.9901	0.9957

Age group <30 is the reference age group. Standard errors (in parentheses) are calculated using the Huber-White correction. P values are in brackets.
*Significant at the P < 0.05 level.
** Significant at the P < 0.01 level.

(conceptual) model, these variables are not found to be significantly different from 0 and thus do not appear to be important in explaining the drop in $\log_{10}$ viral load. Despite their lack of statistical significance, we cannot exclude variables from our model for which we have a conceptual reason to include. Doing so would potentially cause omitted variable bias, another problem discussed in the Violations section.

Analyzing the results from the second equation, which includes the interaction term, we find several differences from the first equation. The interaction between the new drug and baseline viral load, for which we have a conceptual basis, is statistically significant. The effect on viral load of a one-unit increase in baseline viral load on patients who do not receive the new drug is 0.772 (coefficient on baseline viral load). However, the coefficient on the interaction variable indicates that for every one-unit increase in the baseline viral load, the new drug will have an increased effect on the viral load of 0.147. Thus, the overall effect on viral load of a one unit increase in baseline viral load on patients who get the new drug will be 0.147 + 0.772 = 0.919. This tells us that the effect of the new drug is not the same across all baseline viral load levels, but it will be stronger for higher levels of viral load. Notice that by including this interaction term, the new drug variable is no longer significant alone. We also find that while being 45 and older was not significant in the first equation, it is now significant. The coefficient indicates that being 45 and older reduces the $\log_{10}$ viral load by 0.02 relative to the reference category, younger than 30. We now turn to looking at first the properties of the ordinary least squares method, then to violations of some of its most important assumptions.

Properties of the Method of Ordinary Least Squares

OLS has some important statistical properties that make it one of the most powerful methods of regression analysis. These properties comprise the Gauss-Markov theorem. An estimator such as $\hat{\beta}_2$ is referred to as the *best linear unbiased estimator* (BLUE) of β_2 if:

> 1st Property: it is *linear*. The estimator must be a linear function of a random variable.
> 2nd Property: it is *unbiased*. The mean (expected) value, $E(\hat{\beta}_2)$, is equal to the true value, β_2.
> 3rd Property: it has a minimum variance in the class of all such linear unbiased estimators. An unbiased estimator with the least variance is called an *efficient* estimator.

An alternative estimator such as β_2^*, will have a sampling distribution with greater tails (more widespread around the mean value) than that of the ordinary least squares estimator, $\hat{\beta}_2$.

We can now state the Gauss-Markov Theorem: Given the assumptions of the classical linear unbiased regression model, the least-squares estimators, have minimum variance of the class of unbiased estimators, that is, they are blue.

Assumptions of the Method of Ordinary Least Squares

1st Assumption: The expected value of the error is 0.
The mean value of the ε_i , conditional upon the given X_i ,is 0. Referring to Figure 9.1, some of the observations lie above the regression line, so that the ε_i are positive, while other observations lie below the regression line, so that the ε_i are negative. This assumption implies that the positive ε_i offset the negative ε_i , so that the mean of the error term is 0.

2nd Assumption: There is no autocorrelation between the errors.
Autocorrelation implies that the values of ε are correlated. This is a violation of the statistical properties of OLS. If there is autocorrelation, then the parameter estimates will be inefficient. See Kennedy[1] or Gujarati[2] for more information on how to test for and correct for autocorrelation.

3rd Assumption: Homoscedasticity (equal variance of ε_i).
The variance of ε_i for each X_i is some positive constant number equal to σ^2. An example of heteroscedasticity is illustrated in Figure 9.4. Note that as baseline viral load increases the distance between the observation and the line increases. This implies that the variance is larger when

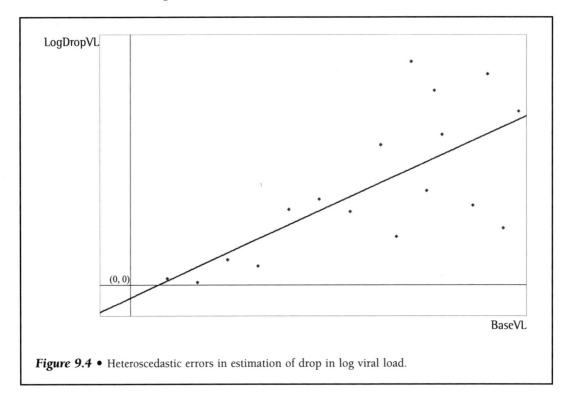

Figure 9.4 • Heteroscedastic errors in estimation of drop in log viral load.

baseline viral load is larger. In the above numerical analysis we used a Huber-White correction for heteroscedasticity. This is a common option in econometric software packages such as Stata. Another possibility is to use generalized or weighted least squares. Please see Kennedy[1] or Gujarati[2] for more information on how to test for and correct for heteroscedasticity.

4th Assumption: The covariance between ε_i and X_i is 0.

This assumption implies that there is no correlation between the error, ε, and the explanatory variable, X. If ε and X are correlated, it is not possible to assess their individual effects on Y. This is one source of a common problem in OLS and one of the most frequently violated assumptions. It is commonly referred to as an endogeneity problem or statistical confounding. The solution to endogeneity is either two-stage least squares or instrumental variables. If panel data are available, fixed effects may be a viable alternative. Please see Kennedy[1] or Gujarati[2] for more information on these alternative estimators.

A test for contemporaneous correlation between the errors and the regressors was introduced in Hausman.[3] When contemporaneous correlation is found to exist, the most common way to deal with it is by using instrumental variables (IV) estimation. IV estimation involves finding an "instrument" for each variable that is contemporaneously correlated with the error. This new independent variable must have two characteristics:

1. It must be uncorrelated with the error.
2. It must be correlated with the independent variable for which it is to serve as an instrument.

Another source of the problem is measurement error. These errors may rise from any source, ranging from hospital coding practices to researchers using the wrong variable as a proxy for something else they wish to measure. Errors in measuring the dependent variable are part of the error term, so that their existence is not a large concern because the independent variables will filter out any correlation. However, when there is error in measuring an independent variable, the fourth assumption of the classical linear model may be violated. These measurement errors make the variable stochastic; in other words, there is an error component associated with the variable. The consequences depend on whether or not the measurement error is distributed independently of the error. That is, if the measurement error is not correlated with the regression error term, then the coefficient may be biased towards 0. As a result, the estimates will be more conservative. However, if measurement error is correlated with the regression error term, the bias can go in either direction, and it is not possible to judge whether the results are conservative or misleading.

5th Assumption: The regression model is specified correctly (there is no specification bias or error).
This may be the most stringent assumption. If important variables are omitted from the model, an incorrect functional form is specified, or the wrong stochastic assumptions are made about the variables, the validity of the estimates may be questionable. If the theory underlying the model is not valid, it is difficult to specify the model correctly. Accordingly, this assumption is important to remind the reader that the results of regression analysis are conditional upon a valid model with the correct variables.

When an important variable is omitted from the estimated model in ordinary least squares, there are three main consequences:

1. The ordinary least squares estimator of the coefficients of the remaining variables may be biased depending on whether the omitted variable is correlated with the other independent variables. If the omitted variable is uncorrelated with the included independent variables, the estimate of the constant term will be biased unless the mean of the omitted variable is 0. The slope coef-ficient estimator remains unbiased. If the omitted variable is correlated with the other variables, then the parameter estimates will always be biased. This is almost always the case.
2. The variance-covariance matrix of β becomes smaller. This result, along with the first, means that omitting a relevant variable can either increase or decrease an estimator's mean square error, depending on the relevant magnitudes of the variance reduction and the bias.
3. The estimator of the now smaller variance-covariance matrix of β is biased upward, because the estimator of σ^2, the variance of the error term, is biased upward. This means that inferences made using these parameters will be inaccurate. This is also true even if the omitted variable is uncorrelated with the other independent variables.

What about the converse? If an irrelevant variable is included? Inclusion of irrelevant variables has two less serious consequences:

1. β and the estimator of its variance-covariance matrix remain unbiased.
2. Unless the irrelevant variable is uncorrelated with the other independent variables, the variance-covariance matrix of β becomes larger, and the ordinary least squares estimator is not as efficient. If this is the case, the mean square error of the estimate is increased.

This often leads to what is commonly known as the "kitchen sink" dilemma of including all possible variables in order to avoid omitted variable bias. The literature recommends using theoretical or conceptual models to guide the specification of the model to be estimated. Tests for misspecification do exist, but there is no unequivocal means of testing for omission of an unknown explanatory variable. This is mainly because other misspecifications, such as incorrect functional form, affect available tests.

Conclusion

Ordinary least squares is probably the most common estimator used in health services research. Indeed, when the assumptions of OLS are met, it is the best linear unbiased estimator of a variable of interest. However, when one or more of the OLS assumptions are violated, alternative techniques are available. Subsequent chapters present and describe these alternative techniques when OLS is no longer appropriate. The next chapter looks at the case in which the dependent variable is dichotomous.

References

1. Kennedy, P. *A Guide to Econometrics*. 4th ed. Malden, MA: Blackwell Publishers Inc.; 1998.
2. Gujarati, D. *Basic Econometrics*. 2nd ed. New York: McGraw-Hill, Inc.; 1988.
3. Hausman, J. 1978. Specification tests in econometrics. *Econometrica*. 46:1251–1272.

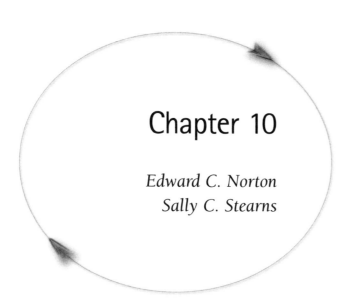

Chapter 10

Edward C. Norton
Sally C. Stearns

Logistic
Regression

The previous chapter provided a solid introduction to linear regression for continuous dependent variables. Dichotomous (dummy) dependent variables are extremely common, however, in health services research and in pharmacoeconomics. Examples include indicators of whether a survey respondent had a hospital admission during the last year, or whether a study participant dies during a clinical trial. Furthermore, many continuous variables are appropriately recoded as dichotomous variables to indicate achieving a meaningful threshold. Examples include whether a patient has an undetectable viral load (rather than a continuous measure of viral load) or whether a baby's birthweight is low (rather than a continuous measure of birthweight).

This chapter provides an introduction to the use and interpretation of the logit model, which is a nonlinear estimation technique frequently used for dichotomous dependent variables. The problems with using ordinary least squares (OLS) for dichotomous dependent variables motivate the use of the logit model. We briefly review the mechanics behind the estimation (maximum likelihood estimation). Then we illustrate the interpretation of the logit model using the same empirical example of a new drug for HIV treatment. We identify several extensions to the basic logit model and conclude by stating the assumptions and properties of maximum likelihood estimation.

Why Not OLS?

It is important to understand that you can use OLS with a dichotomous dependent variable—no statistical package will ever object to such a process. Indeed, using OLS with a dichotomous dependent variable is commonly done, especially in preliminary analysis, for two reasons: (1) the coefficients have an intuitive interpretation—the change in the probability of the event represented by the dependent variable for a one-unit change in the explanatory variable; and (2) the results are generally similar to those from a logit model in terms of the sign and statistical significance of the coefficients, and in terms of the magnitude of the marginal effects around the means of the explanatory variables.

Least squares regression for a dichotomous dependent variable is known as a *linear probability model,* or LPM. The second column of Table 10.1 shows an LPM using the dichotomous dependent variable of whether a study participant's viral load is undetectable. The linear probability model is:

(1) $$\text{Undetectable} = \beta_0 + \beta_1 \text{NewDrug} + \beta_2 \text{BaseVL} + \beta_3 \text{IVDU} + \beta_4 \text{Age30–44} + \beta_5 \text{Age45} + \varepsilon$$

where *Undetectable* is a dichotomous variable equal to 1 when no viral load is found. The explanatory variables are the same as in the regressions in Chapter 9. The interpretation of the coefficient of greatest interest is that receiving the new drug is associated with a 15.7 percentage point increase in the likelihood of having an undetectable viral load, controlling for the baseline value, being an intravenous drug user, and age. The effect is statistically significant ($p < 0.001$, 95% CI of 0.09 to 0.22).

If LPM is so easy to estimate and interpret, then what is the problem? The LPM has three specific problems, each of which are depicted in Figure 10.1. The X's in the figure represent data points. The heavy straight line represents a linear relationship between a continuous explanatory variable and a dichotomous dependent variable. First, although the values of the dependent variable are bounded by 0 and 1 (in fact, they only equal 0 or 1), prediction using the LPM coefficient estimates can yield estimates greater than 1 or less than 0. Such probabilities are impossible. Second, the LPM assumes a linear relationship between the explanatory variable and the dependent variable. Because probabilities are bounded by 0 and 1, however, the marginal effect of a change in an independent variable generally attenuates at extremely high or low values of that independent variable (as shown by the dotted line in Figure 10.1). Third, LPM models are heteroskedastic (i.e., the error term has nonconstant variance), which compromises the validity of the standard errors and statistical tests. The logit model solves the problems of predictions outside the interval and of constant marginal effects by assuming a nonlinear relationship between the independent variables and the dependent variable. The logit model can be estimated with standard errors corrected for heteroscedasticity, thus solving the third problem.

Table 10.1
Estimations Using Dichotomous-Dependent Variable (N = 412)

Variables	LPM β	Logit β	Logistic expβ	Logit with interaction β
Constant	0.967	3.396		4.632
New drug	0.157†	1.532†	4.627†	−2.535
	(0.033)	(0.358)	(1.657)	(2.541)
	[0.001]	[0.001]	[0.001]	[0.319]
Baseline viral load (log base 10)	−0.062†	−0.593*	0.551*	−0.841†
	(0.023)	(0.235)	(0.130)	(0.265)
	[0.007]	[0.011]	[0.011]	[0.002]
IV drug user	0.005	0.102	1.107	0.117
	(0.057)	(0.536)	(0.594)	(0.524)
	[0.929]	[0.849]	[0.849]	[0.822]
Age 30–44	0.133†	0.960†	2.613†	0.936†
	(0.045)	(0.347)	(0.906)	(0.349)
	[0.004]	[0.006]	[0.006]	[0.007]
Age 45+	0.156†	1.271*	3.564*	1.293*
	(0.053)	(0.500)	(1.782)	(0.506)
	[0.003]	[0.011]	[0.011]	[0.011]
New drug × baseline viral load	−	−	−	0.817
	−	−	−	(0.518)
	−	−	−	[0.114]
R-squared	0.0914	−	−	−
Pseudo R-squared	−	0.1175	0.1175	0.1264
Log likelihood	−	−146.1	−146.1	−144.7

All estimations provide robust standard errors in parentheses below the coefficients. The coefficient for the logistic model is the odds ratio. The *p*-values are provided in brackets. The omitted age group is persons <30.
 * $p < 0.05$.
 † $p < 0.01$.

MLE Estimation

Maximum likelihood is a standard method to estimate parameters in nonlinear models. The idea behind maximum likelihood is to choose the set of parameters that makes the probability of observing the data most likely. For example, suppose that you want to estimate the probability that a weighted coin lands heads up when spun. If you spin the weighted coin 100 times, and it lands heads up 40 times, intuition says that the probability *p* that makes this outcome (40 heads and 60 tails) most likely

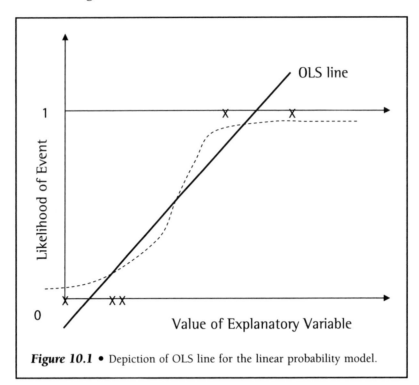

Figure 10.1 • Depiction of OLS line for the linear probability model.

is $p = 0.4$. The likelihood function for this problem is the probability of observing 40 heads and 60 tails, or $L = p^{40}(1 - p)^{60}$. Of all possible values of p between 0 and 1, the value that makes L the largest is 0.4. In summary, although the true probability could be greater or less than 0.4, the best guess given the data is $p = 0.4$.

The logit function $(1 + \exp(-z))^{-1}$ allows the probability of an event p to be a function of many independent variables.

$$(2) \qquad\qquad p = \frac{1}{1 + e^{-(X\beta)}}$$

$$(3) \qquad X\beta = \beta_0 + \beta_1 \text{NewDrug} + \beta_2 \text{BaseVL} + \beta_3 \text{IVDU} + \beta_4 \text{Age30–44} + \beta_5 \text{Age45}$$

Unlike the LPM, the logit function constrains predicted probabilities to be between 0 and 1 for all values of the independent variables.

The likelihood function for a logit model is the product of probabilities, one for each observation. Each probability is a function of covariates. For example, in the HIV data the probability of having an undetectable viral load is

$$(4) \qquad Pr\,(\text{Undetectable}) = \frac{1}{1 + e^{-(\beta_0 + \beta_1 \text{NewDrug} + \beta_2 \text{BaseVL} + \beta_3 \text{IVDU} + \beta_4 \text{Age30–44} + \beta_5 \text{Age45})}}$$

where the β's are the six parameters to be estimated. The likelihood function is the product of 412 terms (one for each observation in the HIV data set) either like the one in Equation 4 or one minus such a term. The maximum likelihood estimators are the set of β's that make the observed outcomes (355 people with undetectable viral load, and 57 with detectable viral load) most likely. Statistical software programs estimate logit models quickly.

Interpretation

The results from the logit model are in many ways similar to the LPM, as seen by comparing the second column of Table 10.1 to the first. Each coefficient's sign, which gives the direction of the relationship between each explanatory variable and the dependent variable, is the same for both estimations. Furthermore, the statistical significance of the relationship for each explanatory variable is roughly the same in the two models, with only small differences in the *p*-values.

With respect to the direction of the effect, the likelihood of having an undetectable viral load is greater for people taking the new drug, for people aged 30 to 44 compared to people under age 30, and for people aged 45 or older compared to people under age 30. All those estimated coefficients are positive. The likelihood of having an undetectable viral load is lower for people with higher baseline levels of viral load (see Magnitude, below). The coefficient for the IV drug user variable is positive in both the LPM and logit models, but because it is not significantly different from zero, changes in the sign of this coefficient would have no meaning in any case.

Magnitude

There are two standard ways to interpret the magnitude of logit coefficients. One way is to convert the logit coefficients to odds ratios by exponentiating each coefficient. Software packages ease conversion by reporting odds ratios instead of coefficients in what is called *logistic regression*. The precise mathematical relationship between the logit and logistic models means that the explanatory power of the two models (as reflected by the pseudo-R^2 or the log likelihood) is exactly the same.

The odds ratio is the ratio of the odds ($p/1 - p$) for two observations that differ only in the value of one independent variable. For example, consider two people who are identical except that one receives the new drug and the other does not. The odds ratio is 4.627 = exp(1.532) (see the fourth column of Table 10.1 for logistic regression results). The odds ratio is 2.61 for a person aged 30 to 44 relative to a person who is less than age 30. The odds ratio for IV drug user is 1.107, although not statistically significantly different from 1.0 (which is the relevant comparison because exp(0) = 1).

The other way to interpret logit coefficients is to compute incremental and marginal effects in terms of percentage point changes, the underlying measure of interest. For illustrative purposes, consider Erica, who has a baseline viral load equal to the sample mean of 4.87, is under 30, is not an IV drug user, and did not receive the new drug. For Erica, the incremental effect of receiving the new drug is the change in probability of an undetectable viral load, holding all else constant. Based on the results in column 3 in Table 10.1, the predicted probability that Erica has an undetectable viral load is

$$0.624 = \frac{1}{1 + e^{-(3.396 - 0.593 \times 4.87)}}$$

If Erica were to take the new drug, her predicted probability would be

$$0.885 = \frac{1}{1 + e^{-(3.396 + 1.532 - 0.593 \times 4.87)}}$$

The new drug increases the probability that Erica has an undetectable viral load by 26 percentage points. This is a 41.7 percent increase ((0.885 − 0.624)/0.624) in the probability of having an undetectable viral load.

Because many researchers are comfortable with the odds ratio interpretation, it is important to explain why the odds ratio can easily be misinterpreted. The odds ratio is often stated as if it were a risk ratio, which it is not. For example, it is incorrect to state that the probability that someone who receives the new drug is 4.627 times more likely to have an undetectable viral load than someone who does not receive the new drug. If the probability of an undetectable viral load is small (less than 5 percent or so), the odds ratio is a reasonable approximation to the risk ratio and is a useful way to present results. However, if the probability of an undetectable viral load is large the two measures differ greatly. The risk ratio for the new drug for Erica is 1.418 = 0.885/0.624, meaning that taking the drug results in a 41.8 percent increase in probability of undetectable viral load. This is far less than a four-fold increase, the incorrect interpretation of an odds ratio greater than 4.0.

The marginal effect of a continuous variable can be computed two ways. The first is analogous to an incremental effect. Compute probabilities for two cases that differ only in the value of a continuous variable. For example, consider a change in the logarithm of the baseline viral load from the mean of 4.87 to 5.87. The probability of having an undetectable viral load for Erica is then

$$0.479 = \frac{1}{1 + e^{-(3.396 + 1.532 - 0.593 \times 5.87)}}$$

The marginal effect of baseline viral load is –0.145 = 0.479 – 0.624. In other words, this means that for someone like Erica, an increase in the baseline viral load of a factor of 10 (a one-unit change in the logarithm of baseline viral load) leads on average to a decrease in the probability of an undetectable viral load of nearly fifteen percentage points. The marginal effect can also be approximated by multiplying the coefficient for the variable of interest β_x by the predicted probability p multiplied by 1 minus the probability $\beta_x \times p \times (1 - p)$, where p depends on all the explanatory variables. The marginal effect of baseline viral load is –0.139 = –0.593 × 0.624 × (1 – 0.624).

Unlike a linear probability model, a logit model implicitly assumes that the marginal effect of a continuous explanatory variable is not constant. Instead, the marginal effect depends on the predicted probability. It is relatively small when the predicted probability is close to either zero or one, and relatively large when the predicted probability is close to one half. The marginal effect is the slope of the dashed line in Figure 10-1. For example, consider Rachel, who is like Erica in all ways except age. Rachel is more than 45 years old. The probability that Rachel has an undetectable viral load is 0.856. The incremental effect of the new drug for Rachel is only 11 percentage points, and the marginal effect of baseline viral load is only negative seven percentage points. Because Erica's predicted probability is closer to one half than Rachel's, the incremental and marginal effects are larger for Erica than for Rachel.

Interaction Terms

Interaction effects are more complicated to interpret in logit models than in linear models. Neither the sign nor the magnitude of the interaction effect can be determined by looking only at the coefficient on the interaction term.[1,2] Nor can the statistical significance of the interaction term be determined simply by the statistical significance of the coefficient on the interaction term. Furthermore, the odds ratio interpretation of logit results is not correct for variables with interacted terms. The estimated coefficient on an interacted term in a logistic regression is the ratio of odds ratios, and, therefore, extremely hard to interpret.

The full interaction effect—how a change in *both* interacted variables affects the predicted probability—requires either computing the double derivative of the logit function with respect to both variables or computing a double difference. This issue is beyond the scope of this text. For more details, see References.

Statistical Significance

The standard statistical test for hypothesis testing after running a logit model is a z-test (or Wald test), not a t-test, as in linear regression. The z-test, however, is analogous to a t-test. Asymptotic theory for maximum likelihood estimation states that the estimated parameters are asymptotically normal. To test the statistical significance of one parameter, divide the estimated parameter by its standard error. If the estimated parameter divided by its standard error is more than 1.96 in absolute value, then the parameter is statistically significant at the 5-percent level. For example, in the logit model the coefficient on new drug is 1.532, and its standard error (controlling for heteroscedasticity) is 0.358. Therefore, the z-statistic is 4.28, which is highly statistically significant. The 95% confidence interval is [0.830, 2.234].

Some statistical software report the related Wald statistic, which is simply the square of the estimated parameter divided by its variance. The 5 percent critical value is $3.84 = 1.96^2$. Wald tests can be used to test more complicated hypotheses about multiple coefficients. Wald tests account for heteroscedasticity.

As explained earlier, the LPM model suffers from heteroscedasticity (nonconstant variance), and the basic logit model also has this problem. Therefore, it is generally recommended to estimate robust standard errors, as was done in Table 10.1. Robust standard errors ensure valid confidence intervals and statistical tests even in the presence of heteroscedasticity. Most statistical packages easily compute robust standard errors for logit models. The differences in the standard errors or p-values are usually minor. For example, nonrobust standard errors for the logit model in Table 10.1 are slightly smaller (and, therefore, the p-values are slightly higher) for the coefficients for the new drug, baseline viral load, and age 45 or older variables. Yet it is prudent to use the robust standard errors to ensure that the statistical tests are appropriate.

Goodness of Fit Measures

As discussed in the previous chapter, the coefficient of variation R^2 is the most commonly used measure of goodness of fit for linear regression, largely because it has the intuitively appealing definition of representing the proportion of the variance in the dependent variable explained by the model. Unfortunately, R^2 is not defined for logit models, although several different methods of calculating an analogous measure of goodness of fit have been proposed. Some of these, which are often called pseudo-R^2 statistics, involve calculations using the log likelihood of the estimated model relative to the log likelihood from a model including only a constant term. The value of 0.1175 calculated for the model in column 3 is calculated using one of these formulas. Logit models rarely have high pseudo-R^2 statistics.

One alternative that some people recommend is to round the predicted values from the model up to 1 or down to 0 (based on whether the predicted value is greater or less than 0.5) and then calculate the percent of rounded predictions that match the actual value in the sample. The problem with this approach is that models with a dependent variable that has a mean close to 0 or 1 will seem to predict well, even if none of the explanatory variables are statistically significant. This approach is not recommended.

Related Models and Extensions

Probit

The *probit* model is a common alternative to the logit model in some disciplines when the dependent variable is dichotomous. The probit model assumes that the error term has a normal distribution instead of a logistic distribution. However, these two distributions are nearly identical, and the assumption of one or the other is not testable in practice. The choice is largely a matter of taste. The estimated coefficients from a logit model are roughly 1.6 times those from a probit. Signs and statistical significance are usually the same. The probit model does not have an odds ratio interpretation. However, it is closely related to the *ordered probit*, *tobit*, *random effects probit*, and *Heckman selection* models. The *complementary log-log* model is an asymmetric alternative to the logit and probit models. This model is used primarily when the outcome of interest is rare.

Extensions to the Logit Model

When the dependent variable is categorical and ordered, neither least squares regression nor logit are appropriate. Examples of categorical ordered dependent variables include self-reported health status (excellent, good, fair, poor) or birthweight, with thresholds for very low birthweight (<1500 g), low birthweight (1500–2500 g), and normal birthweight. The *ordered logit* model allows covariates to change the predicted probability of being in each category without making arbitrary assumptions about the distance between the categories on a linear scale as one does when running a linear regression.

When the dependent variable is categorical but not ordered, the ordered logit model is not appropriate. Examples include dependent variables representing the type of treatment (drug A, drug B, or drug C) or choice of college major (humanities, social sciences, or engineering). The *multinomial logit* model allows the explanatory variables to influence the probability of each choice. One implicit assumption of the multinomial logit is that adding or deleting choices to the dependent variable will not change the relative probability of choice among the remaining categories. This assumption, known as the independence from irrelevant alternatives (IIA), is often violated. For example, imagine modeling the choice of presidential candidates Bush, Gore, and Nader. If Nader dropped out of the race and Bush and Gore were neck-and-neck, would it be reasonable to assume that those who would have voted for Nader would instead roughly split their votes between the remaining candidates? Probably not; hence, IIA is violated in this example. More computationally complex models, such as the *nested logit* model and *multinomial probit* model, relax the IIA assumption but are hard to estimate.

When there are repeated observations on groups, the *conditional logit* model can eliminate unobserved group fixed effects. This model, however, places fairly heavy demands on the data. Only groups with both positive and negative outcomes remain in the model, so short panels may lose most of their observations.

MLE Assumptions and Properties

The assumptions needed for MLE are highly technical and not illuminating. Suffice it to say that the likelihood function needs to be smooth enough to take multiple derivatives and to compute Taylor series. These assumptions are not a problem for standard logit regression models.

MLE has nice statistical properties. MLE is consistent, asymptotically normal, and efficient. *Consistent* means that as the sample size grows, the estimated parameters will get arbitrarily close to the true values. *Asymptotically normal* means that as the sample size grows, the estimated parameters have a normal distribution. Therefore, normal statistical theory provides the basis for hypothesis tests about coefficients. Unlike linear regression models that use t-tests for hypothesis testing of single coefficients, MLE uses z-tests (for normal distributions) because the coefficients are asymptotically normal. *Asymptotically efficient* means that no other consistent and asymptotically normal estimator has a smaller asymptotic variance.

Suggested Reading

Woolridge JM. *Introductory Economics: A Modern Approach.* 2nd ed. Mason, WI: Thompson-Southwestern; 2003.

References

1. Ai C, Norton EC. Interaction terms in logit and probit models. *Economics Letters.* 2003;80(1):123–129.

2. Norton EC, Wang H, Ai C. Computing interaction effects and standard errors in logit and probit models. *Stata J.* 2004;4(2):103–116.

Section Four

Integrative Models

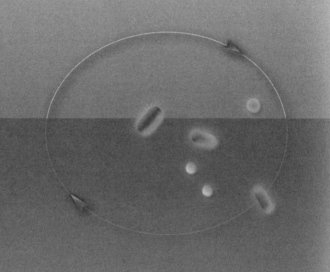

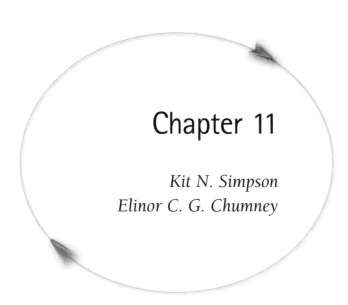

Chapter 11

Kit N. Simpson
Elinor C. G. Chumney

Decision Analysis Models

Introduction

An integrative or stochastic decision model can be an extremely useful tool to reach beyond the limits of the data that researchers have collected in an attempt to the answer important questions facing decision makers.[1] Data from clinical, pharmacoeconomic, or outcomes research studies are often incomplete, because of both the enormous number of resources involved and the need to quickly document the clinical effects of interventions. As a result, studies can be limited in both the breadth of data collected and the length of time patients are followed. Patients in clinical trials, for example, are routinely observed for short-term marker or surrogate endpoints such as blood pressure reductions, rather than long-term outcomes such as strokes avoided. Decision models are frequently used to predict long-term effects and multidimensional outcomes based on actual data on fewer variables observed for a shorter time period.[2] In the absence of direct primary empirical data to address key issues, the use of modeling to estimate effectiveness and cost-effectiveness is considered to be a valid form of scientific inquiry.[3]

Decision models structure a clinical problem mathematically, allowing researchers to enumerate the health outcomes and costs expected from using competing treatments. They integrate data and information from many sources under a clearly specified set of assumptions and are useful for informing discussions for and against specific policy choices. Traditionally, researchers have structured clinical problems by either summarizing the major treatment choices and their resulting outcomes in a decision tree (also called a probability tree) or describing the disease process as a series of health states that patients have a specific probability of experiencing over time (a state-transition or Markov model).

Decision tree models represent a sequence of treatment decisions and probabilistic health outcomes over time in a series of chance and decision nodes. They are an extremely useful tool for representing relatively simple disease and treatment processes in deciding on a best course of action. However as we will discuss later in this chapter, one limitation of decision tree models is that they are not well suited to representing events that recur over time.

Because Markov models or state-transition models are designed to allow for event recurrence, they have eclipsed decision tree models in popularity for more complicated and chronic diseases such as HIV. Markov models depict the natural history of disease as a sequence of mutually exclusive health states, defined to capture important clinical traits such as acute event history. They also make the assumption that patients assigned to a given health state incur similar economic costs and enjoy a comparable quality of life. They then use what is known about the population, the disease, and the effect of interventions to govern the transitions into and out of the various health states.[4]

Using Modeling Studies

Modeling studies may be useful for informing decisions at many stages of a drug's development. Simple early modeling efforts performed prior to Phase I or II clinical trials can help identify key relationships between factors that influence the efficacy and cost of care. They can also predict the sample size necessary to detect statistical significance regarding health-related quality of life or cost measures. Most importantly, such models can be used to inform judgments about the cost-effectiveness ratio for a new compound compared to drugs in current use given several pricing assumptions. This may be quite important if current drugs are relatively cheap but have low efficacy, and new compounds are expected to be both more expensive to manufacture and more efficacious.

Modeling studies that are based on data from Phase III or IV trials may have many different purposes, and their designs must vary to reflect such differences. Phase III or IV models are often used to translate efficacy results from trial data into estimates of effectiveness expected for patients under usual practice conditions. Such models may link "marker" or surrogate endpoints (e.g., CD4 cell changes) to epidemiological measures of disease, such as rates of expected opportunistic events for AIDS patients.[5] Alternatively, they may simply translate differences in resource use and outcomes reported from clinical studies into incremental cost effectiveness ratios, given specific assumptions about practice patterns, cost of resources, or country of use. Modeling may also be used to examine expected differences for subgroups of patients, for different comparators (including other technologies, such as surgery), or for specific types of populations, such as members of a managed care group. Most importantly, models may be used to estimate the expected lifetime costs and effects from trial results that are limited to data collected over a fairly short time period.

Linking Data

As noted earlier, models may be used to predict long-term effects based on actual data from a more limited time period. Because of both the large number of resources involved and the need to document meaningful clinical effects quickly, clinical trial data often cover only a limited period of time; patients are observed for short-term marker or surrogate endpoints such as blood pressure reduction rather than long-term outcomes such as strokes avoided or early death. By contrast, observational data (e.g., epidemiological or billing databases) follow patients for extended periods of time and allow researchers to document the long-term health implications of the surrogate endpoints.

When short-term clinical trial data are linked with observational or other types of data reflecting long-term outcomes and resource use, researchers must be careful to assure that these data could have come from two (or more) samples of the same population. Essentially, they must document that the incorporated data sets are similar with respect to both health risks and the propensity for resource use. To do this, researchers rely on analyses of linkage variables that predict either critical outcomes or specific levels of resource use. This is often the most difficult part of modeling and the one most open to challenges from critics.

Linkage variables always include some demographic or disease-related variables that were originally used to exclude patients from enrollment in a trial. Second-level linkage variables encompass systems that classify acute episodes, such as *International Classification of Diseases,* 9th edition (ICD9), or *Physicians' Current Procedural Terminology,* 4th edition (CPT4), codes for the episodes of care. Severity of illness indices, explaining either disease stage complexity or the prevalence of comorbid conditions, may also be used to link data sets for modeling. One of the most commonly used indices, especially in critical care, is the Acute Physiology and Chronic Health Evaluation (APACHE) score. Finally outcome measures, such as being discharged in a dependent state (either with home health care or to a nursing home setting) may be used to control for differences in resource use and outcomes at the end of acute disease episodes.

The following issues should be considered when clinical and observational data are used together. First, the quality of coding in observational or billing data may be quite inferior to the coding or diagnostic descriptions found in clinical trial data. Observational data may be "dirty," with invalid observations or more than one observation for each patient. It may also be systematically biased in the selection of disease codes, having a high prevalence of codes for which reimbursement is favorable, and few codes for cases with poor payment rules. Clinical trial data have limitations as well, as clinical episodes may be artificially mild because adverse developments are recognized early through careful monitoring. It may also be biased, in that the codes of particular interest to investigators may appear more often than would be expected in regular practice. Finally, both the clinical and observational data may be biased against the inclusion of specific types of patients. For example, wealthier patients may be excluded from Medicaid databases and people without a telephone may be excluded from surveys based on random digit telephone dialing.

Data Sources

Numerous data sources have been used to supplement clinical trial data for modeling, but most of them have serious limitations that must be considered in an analysis. Hospital discharge data are commonly used to furnish data on episodes of acute illnesses. These data may seem standardized, but may actually exclude severe "charity" cases. The quality of coding in these types of data also may vary; some conditions may be reported in a very high proportion of cases while others may regularly be excluded.

Furthermore, hospital discharge data do not contain information on care provided by physicians, and most lack information on drugs used. It is also important to note that the monetary values reported reflect billing charges, not costs of care. Some observational data represent medical practice patterns that are atypical (HMO data are among this group). Insurance billing data are often "right-hand censored" because patients lose eligibility if they lose their job. Medicare data must be used with caution for patients in specific age groups, because of the age-dependent eligibility criteria for these programs.

Whenever observational or epidemiological data are used to supplement clinical trial data for the purpose of modeling effectiveness or costs, one must keep in mind that these data will be assumed in the model to come from one population. It is, therefore, often necessary to perform direct or indirect adjustments on one of the data sets so that the important linkage variables are prevalent in the same proportion in both data sets. Multivariate statistical analysis or survival analysis may also be used to adjust estimates for biasing factors. Even the best analyst, however, cannot exclude the possibility that important unmeasured or unknown factors are confounding the data.

Sensitivity Analysis

Models are only as good as the assumptions and the data that are used for their construction. Decision makers, therefore, need some reassurance that predictions are not completely irrelevant to informing decisions. There are two ways to provide some assurance about the validity of modeling results: model validation and model sensitivity analysis.

Models need to have face validity, that is, they must seem reasonable to individuals who have expert knowledge in the clinical area of specialization. Models should also have predictive validity; they should be able to predict the prevalence of key conditions and costs for populations other than those on which they were designed. Unfortunately, complete data on cost and outcomes for similar populations, or even for the therapies that are being modeled, are rare. In such cases researchers must rely on sensitivity analyses.

Sensitivity analyses test a model's response to variations in the levels of parameters of variables included. It answers the "what if" questions. Although parameter values are usually entered into the model as discrete values, they may be drawn from a range of potential values (i.e., a confidence interval) based on random chance or the approach to measuring. Moreover, practitioners and researchers may want to adapt the model results to slightly different populations or scenarios than those used in a model. To test the effect of these variations on the model results, the value of a single parameter may be replaced with ones that are less likely, but still possible. For example, these could include values at the limits of the parameter's confidence interval or best/worst case scenario values. This is an example of one-way sensitivity analysis.

For a two-way sensitivity analysis, the values of two parameters are changed simultaneously. The stability of model predictions may also be tested by randomly varying many of the key parameter values within their confidence intervals. This type of testing may be done using a second order Monte Carlo approach provided in several of the commercially available modeling software programs.

If these extreme valuations do not affect the model's estimates enough to change the policy conclusion, then the model is characterized as stable or robust. Otherwise the model is recognized as sensitive to changes in the given parameters, and this can be taken into consideration in decisions. The value of the parameter at which the model yields a different conclusion in the sensitivity test is known as the threshold value.

Decision Trees

Decision trees depict what may be expected to happen to a group of patients who receive different treatments. Each treatment choice is organized as one major branch originating from a central point, called a decision node. The population for each branch is then grouped into subgroups by:

1. The process of care common to patients, and
2. The intermediate and final outcomes experienced by patients over an episode of the illness.

Figure 11.1 illustrates how a decision tree may be employed to use efficacy data from clinical trials to compare expected outcomes for a new drug to usual care for a cohort of 200 patients.

Convention dictates that choices in therapy are represented by square decision nodes and probability distributions are represented by round nodes, with the proportion of patients who fall into a group indicated below each branch, and the type of group written above the branch. For example, in Figure 11.1, the probability of being treated in the hospital is 20% for each type of therapy, but the probability of being discharged well is 90% for hospitalized patients who receive the new drug and 80% for those patients receiving usual care. The average cost of care for a group is given at the end of each branch, as is the length of the illness episode. The total cost for each kind of therapy is then calculated by multiplying all conditional probabilities along the branches and then multiplying the resulting probabilities by the average cost indicated for each branch. This is called "rolling back" the decision tree.

To roll back the decision tree for Figure 11.1, we would first assume that we have a population of 100 patients each taking the new drug or receiving usual care. We could then calculate the cost associated with the top branch (branch 1) by multiplying the number of patients taking the new drug (100) by the probability they are hospitalized (20%), then multiplying that quantity by the probability the hospitalized patients on the new drug are discharged well (0.90), and finally multiplying that quantity by the cost associated with that experience ($10,000). The average cost per treated case on the new drug could then be calculated and compared against the average cost of usual care as follows:

New drug: $180,000 for branch 1 = 100 × 0.20 × 0.90 × $10,000
$30,000 for branch 2 = 100 × 0.20 × 0.10 × $15,000
$14,400 for branch 3 = 100 × 0.80 × 0.90 × $200
+ $6,400 for branch 4 = 100 × 0.80 × 0.10 × $800
$230,800 total (an average of $2,308 per case treated)

Usual care: $157,600 for branch 1 = 100 × 0.20 × 0.80 × $9,850
$60,000 for branch 2 = 100 × 0.20 × 0.20 × $15,000
$3,200 for branch 3 = 100 × 0.80 × 0.80 × $50
+ $9,600 for branch 4 = 100 × 0.80 × 0.20 × $600
$230,400 total (an average of $2,304 per case treated)

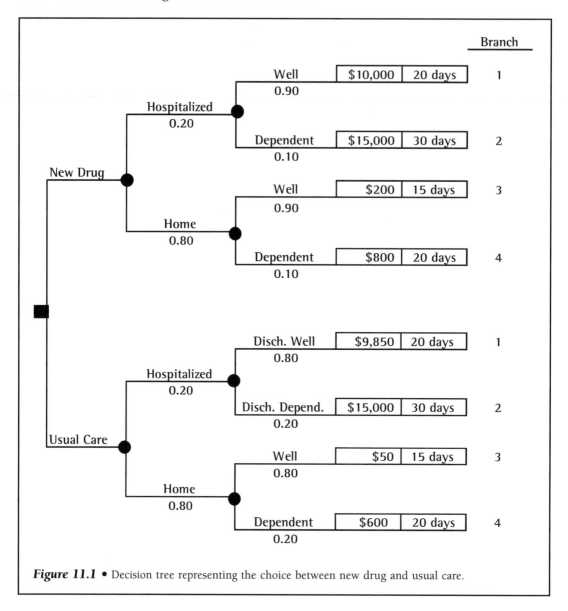

Figure 11.1 • Decision tree representing the choice between new drug and usual care.

This cost comparison analysis shows that, from the perspective of a health care system, it would cost $4 more in direct medical care costs per case for the new drug than for usual care. We can also calculate morbidity days, simply by using the sick days at each terminal nodes instead of the costs in each calculation; doing so reveals a total of 1,660 days lost to illness for the 100 patients on the new drug and 1,720 days lost to illness for those receiving usual care.

The costs vary with the perspective. For example, costs are calculated differently if the researcher is examining the issue from an employer's perspective rather than the medical care system perspective. If all patients are assumed to be working adults, and their employer has to hire temporary staff at a new cost of $50 per day of absence, then rolling back the tree while including the employer's cost per morbidity day (direct medical care and other direct costs) reveals that patients treated with the new drug had an average of 16.6 days absence from work, while patients treated with usual care had an average of 17.2 days absence. At a net cost for temporary help of $50 per day, the total cost per episode to an employer is $26 less for a patient treated with the new drug ($3,138 compared to $3,164 for usual treatment).

If instead the researcher wanted to compare a new drug and usual care from the perspective of the medical care system (the perspective that is most often used), he would want to consider the cost of medical resources used and any differences in morbidity suffered by an average patient. One hundred patients treated with the new drug will lose a total of 1,660 days to illness, while the 100 patients treated with usual care are expected to lose 1,720 days being sick, or a difference of 60 days and $400, giving a cost-effectiveness ratio of $6.67 per morbidity day avoided.

If patients hate being sick and value each day at only 50% of a day without illness, then the patients treated with the new drug gain the value of 0.5 days in full health for each of the 60 days of morbidity avoided, or 30 quality adjusted days, at a cost to the medical care system of $400. When this is reported as cost per quality adjusted life year (QALY), the convention for cost utility analyses (CUA), the cost utility ratio for new drug therapy is very reasonable at $4,867 per QALY compared to most current treatments.[1]

As illustrated above, a decision tree is a useful organizing framework for calculating the different types of outcomes that would be expected for acute events under different treatment assumptions and costing perspectives. Although decision trees can be used to inform many clinical and management decisions in health care, published papers using decision trees often focus on comparing emerging clinical or preventive health interventions at a time when the evidence for a new intervention is sparse. In such cases, a decision analysis can combine the limited new efficacy data available with disease history, epidemiological, and cost data to estimate differences in expected outcomes under a clearly articulated set of assumptions. While the results of this type of analysis do not provide clear evidence either for or against the adoption of a new therapy, it often provides an invaluable framework for policy discussions, and nearly always increases our understanding of the key factors that are associated with the desired outcomes from a particular therapy.[6]

An example of the use of a decision tree very early in the chain of evidence collection is illustrated in the paper by Marshall and colleagues[7] investigating the potential of a new method for screening high risk patients for lung cancer. In this policy paper, the authors used one year follow-up data from the first 1,000 patients to receive a helical computed tomography scan (HCT) to detect early lung cancer. Randomized clinical trials of screening for lung cancer in the U.S. in the 1970s using chest x-ray and sputum cytology failed to demonstrate an impact on mortality, and screening has since been discouraged by cancer societies and health care task forces. However, in 1999 Henschke and colleagues published a case series indicating a substantial "left stage shift" in lung cancer cases found through HCT.[8] This finding created new possibilities for detecting and treating lung cancer earlier and with greater success. A decision tree (Figure 11.2) was used to estimate the potential benefits and costs from screening for lung cancer under specific assumptions. Marshall and colleagues combined the results from the baseline screening published by the Henschke group with data from the SEER national cancer registry database to estimate the potential survival improvements, using Medicare cancer cost data to estimate the economic impacts expected if screening with HCT became current practice. The authors reported three major insights delivered by the decision model. Under the assumptions specified in the model: (1) a one-time prevalence screen for lung cancer with HCT scanning in a high-risk cohort of 60–74 years of age appears cost-effective at $5,940/LY; (2) the model estimates are sensitive to the prevalence of lung cancer in the screening population (a decrease from 2.7% to 0.7% in assumed lung cancer prevalence increased the CER to $22,629/LY); and (3) the amount of lead time bias assumed in the model was critical (a 1-year lead time bias assumption increased the CER to $58,183/LY, and the model could not identify health benefits if lead time bias was assumed to be greater than about 1.5 years). This last finding made it clear that evidence on the magnitude of lead time bias for lung cancer was needed before population screening programs outside of clinical trials should be seriously considered. When evaluating the effectiveness of the early detection and treatment of a condition, the lead time (the period between early detection of disease and the time of its usual clinical presentation) must be subtracted from the overall survival time of screened patients to avoid lead time bias. Otherwise early detection merely increases the duration of the patients' awareness of their disease without reducing their mortality or morbidity. This modeling effort is an excellent example of how the results of a decision analysis may help focus the attention of the scientific community on the key factors that must be better illuminated before a new intervention is implemented.

Markov–Type Decision Models

A Markov or state-transition decision analysis model structure is used to organize the data for conditions where patients' health experience can be defined as a progression through different disease stages. Each stage in a Markov-type model is defined as a health state, and it may be possible to progress through stages of increasing severity, as well as from very severe stages to less severe stages, or even to be cured. Markov models are especially useful for predicting long-term outcomes such as survival when clinical trial results use intermediate health outcomes or surrogate markers such as CD4 cell counts to measure the clinical efficacy, effectiveness, and safety of treatments for complex chronic conditions. Markov-type structures are often used for modeling in cases where a decision tree would have a large number of sub-branches that are nearly identical except for differences in their preceding probability nodes. Thus, a Markov-type structure may be used to simplify very "bushy" decision trees.

Markov models are especially useful for examining outcome differences for new treatments for conditions that have clearly differentiated health states.[9] These states can be defined by (1) prognosis,

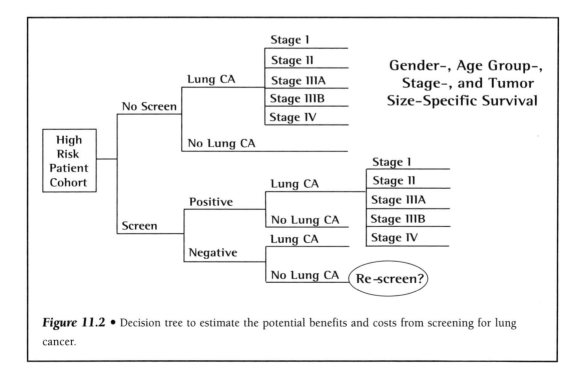

Figure 11.2 • Decision tree to estimate the potential benefits and costs from screening for lung cancer.

such as in cancer stages A, B, C, and D; (2) standardized characteristics of the condition, such CDC stages A, B, or C for patients with HIV disease; or (3) by combinations of laboratory test values that have been shown to be prognostic; such as different levels of CD4 counts and RNA viral load measured in patients with HIV disease. Sometimes we can observe changes in structures used for decision models for a condition as our understanding of the condition affects the endpoints acceptable for clinical trials, since the linkage between reported trial results and epidemiological data is an important factor for selecting the structural framework for a decision model.

This relationship is readily observed in the AIDS models that have been published in the last 15 years. The efficacy measures in the early trials of antiretroviral drugs were progression from asymptomatic HIV disease to AIDS or death, and early models used simple decision trees or state-transition models with few health states based on AIDS and death. As CD4 cell counts became a routinely reported measure of immune deficiency and RNA viral load began to be considered a strong indicator of the risk of disease progression, the health states used in the published decision models of treatments for HIV disease became defined by these markers. Furthermore, as our understanding of HIV disease progressed and our medical armamentarium increased, published HIV disease models progressed to using Markov-type structures with many health states, even linking sequential state-transition structures to capture the complexity of a condition which was transforming from a rapidly fatal disease to a severe chronic illness requiring lifelong monitoring and therapy. The AIDS modeling papers by Schulman et al. (1991),[12] Simpson et al. (1994),[2] Chancellor et al. (1997),[10] Freedberg et al. (2001),[13] and Simpson et al. (2004)[14] illustrate this progression.

In a state-transition or Markov model, the disease process is carved into time periods of equal length defined by a set of health states. Each health state has a specific average quality of life, risk of progression or cure, and expected cost. The progression for a specific group of patients is then defined by the length of time they spend in each health state. Some health states are final or absorbing, meaning that once a patient reaches this state no further progression or improvement will occur. Death is always an absorbing health state, but other states, such as cured or "surgical removal of . . . ." may also be defined as absorbing states if they are assumed to happen no more than once to any one individual. Each health state lasts for a specific time period (1 hour, day, week, month, or year); this is called the length of a cycle in the model. The choice of length for a cycle will depend on the length of the illness episode modeled, the length of time included in the efficacy and epidemiological data available, and the average time included in cost data which are usually reported as aggregates. The choice of a model cycle time is an optimization process. The objective is to find the longest time period that fits the majority of the patients' natural disease episodes, the efficacy data, and the cost data, while making sure that the model does not inadvertently exclude differential outcomes for patients with very short episodes of care. Estimates for patient groups with very long episodes of care can be accommodated by having patients occupy a health state for more than one cycle. Thus, the selection of cycle length is often more of an art than a science.

Once a model's health states and cycle times have been defined, the available data can be analyzed to populate the model. Two types of data are needed: parameters and transition probabilities. Parameters are mean values for measures of interest that are specific to each health state. For example, an AIDS Markov model would use parameters that accounted for the mean risk of getting an AIDS event, mean cost of treating an average AIDS event, and mean quality of life weight (utility) that patients assign to living in that health state.

Transition probabilities are similar to the probability nodes in the decision tree. They function like gates between connected health states. Each transition probability defines the proportion of patients in a current health state who are allowed to move to another state once the cycle time has been completed. For example, the transition probability of moving from health state A to health state B is the percent of individuals who would progress from health state A to health state B during the time of one model cycle under the treatment conditions that are tested in the model. This seems simple, but getting these data can be complicated because the standard epidemiological measures of risk, such as relative risk or odds ratios, account for the overall risk of disease progression across health states included in a model, not the contingent risk of progression from one health state to another, which is what we need in order to calculate transition probabilities. These transition probabilities are the critical variables that contain the differences in efficacy between the therapies compared in the model. They are the "engine" that drives the population through the model at different rates for different treatments. Getting the model transition probabilities right, and especially getting the differences in transition probabilities right for the treatments compared in a Markov model, is the most critical aspect of designing a Markov model. The effects of even small variations in the transition probability differences often swamp the effects of relatively large differences in parameter values for cost, events, or quality of life in most models. This characteristic of Markov models is often not recognized by reviewers of modeling papers who have not been trained in modeling.

The probabilities of moving from health state A to health state B during a model cycle, as well as the probability of moving from state B to state A, are entered into a table called a transition matrix. This table has one row and one column for each health state. Thus, a transition matrix for a model with five health states will have five rows and five columns, with a total of 25 cells. In a Markov model where patients can move from any one state to any other state at the end of each cycle, all 25 cells must contain an accurate contingent probability of a patient's move from one health state to the next. A Markov model with 10 health states, which allows movement between all health states, requires $10 \times 10 = 100$ contingent probability calculations. If we need at least 30 observations for each calculation (a good rule of thumb for such calculations), such a model would require a minimum of 3,000 patient observations to populate the transition matrix. Given that the value of a decision modeling study is to inform discussions before much efficacy data is available, is easy to see the virtue of keeping the number of model health states low and making as many simplifying assumptions as possible to disallow movements between some model health states.

Once the health states and cycle times have been specified, and the transitions and parameters calculated, the model can be programmed. Markov models can be solved as mathematical equations using matrix algebra, they can be executed with spreadsheet software using one column for each health state and one row for each cycle, or they can be programmed in special software, such as TreeAge.

Our preference is to program the models in Excel because this approach is easy and transparent, allowing the observation of patients moving through the model. Furthermore, executing a Markov model in spreadsheet software allows researchers to examine and output aggregates of any parameter of interest at a specific time period. Thus they can create graphs that illustrate the flow of funds, cost and use of specific resources, such as drugs, or the time at which specific benchmarks are reached, such as median survival. The Markov models used by Chancellor and colleagues[10] and the one described by Simpson et al.[11] provide examples of a relatively simple and a more complex use of the Markov modeling structure, as we will see.

Use of Markov Models for HIV Disease

Markov models have been widely used to examine the cost-effectiveness or cost consequences of antiretroviral therapy, prophylaxis treatment, or screening in HIV/AIDS.[11] Markov approaches are especially well-suited to model the progression of HIV/AIDS and typically contain health states that are defined by CD4 cell counts and viral load. These health states are associated with transition probabilities that are derived from information in the published literature based on epidemiological studies and prior clinical trials. Markov models assume that transition probabilities are dependent only upon the immediately previous health state; thus transition probabilities can be derived from existing literature independent from the actual study time in which they occurred. The proportion of patients in each health state that will have an AIDS defining event can then be projected with its subsequent resource utilization and costs.

The model described by Chancellor[11] is a fairly simple example of a Markov structure applied to HIV disease. It has three transitional health states which define an increasing deterioration in a patient's immune system; A is asymptomatic, B is asymptomatic but with a low CD4 cell count, and C is AIDS; its one absorbing health state, D, is death. The cycle time in the model is 1 year. At the end of each cycle patients can (1) stay in their current health state, (2) move to any other health state with a worse immune status, or (3) die. No improvements are allowed in the model. Thus, the transition matrix should have four rows and four columns, or 16 cells. Six of these cells are empty (with a value of 0), the one indicating state D moving to state D (death) would be 1.0, and the rest have actual annual transition rates derived from epidemiological data. Costs were assigned to each health state based on the average annual costs recorded for patients in large observational databases in each health state.

If we compare the structure and parameters used in the Chancellor model which was published in 1997 to those used in the model published by Simpson and colleagues in 2004,[11] we discover that the later model uses a far more complex Markov structure. It has 13 health states, including death, the absorbing state. Its health states are defined by combinations of values of CD4 cell counts and RNA viral load, it includes a utility adjustment to reflect differences in health-related quality of life for each health state, and it is not limited to capturing differences between two initial antiretroviral therapies because it carries these differences out to capture any differences which would exist for a second or third regimen.

Over a period of only 7 years it appears that we are seeing an order of magnitude increase in the complexity and data requirements for an AIDS model. The number of cells in the transition matrix has increased from 16 in the Chancellor model to 169 in the Simpson model. We are no longer considering just the two drug treatments of interest, but also subsequent therapies. Finally, the health states in the model are defined by combinations of two laboratory measures, not by the CDC stage definition for HIV disease, and an adjustment for differences in quality of life for each health state has been incorporated in the model.

These differences between the two models are not simply the result of differences of opinion between the two modeling groups on how best to operationalize a Markov model for HIV disease, they are dictated by the change in practice patterns and the growth in the scientific knowledge of HIV disease which has occurred in the 7-years interim. The redefinition of the health states was needed because clinical trials today report efficacy differences in terms of viral load suppression and CD4 cell gains. The large increase in the number of health states was required to enable the model to capture the fact that competing drug regimens may have the same efficacy for patients who have a relatively normal immune function, but have very different levels of efficacy for patients who are severely immune compromised. The addition of quality of life adjustments to the model reflects the fact that research in the years between the design of the two models found that some HIV drug regimens have low severity side effects, such as nausea, diarrhea, head ache, that their survival benefit is nearly lost due to these negative impacts on quality of life. Lastly, research in the last 7 years has clearly shown that the HIV-virus becomes resistant to specific drug cocktails over time, and that some new drug regimens are better at suppressing resistant virus than others. Thus, it is no longer sufficient to capture the effects of the current drug treatments; a sensitive model must also be able to reflect differences in the level of resistance conferred to the virus once the current regimen has failed. This is only possible if the model extends beyond one regimen.

These two modeling papers each employed a Markov structure as an organizing framework, they were both programmed in Excel, and they based they their transition probabilities and cost estimates on archival epidemiological and cost data from large observational patient cohorts. However, they used different definitions of health states and had vastly different levels of complexity. It would not be appropriate to use the Chancellor model to estimate differences in outcomes for the new drugs that are currently under development. This model reflects a set of assumptions which were acceptable in 1997, but which are too simple given the scientific knowledge of HIV disease that we have today. Yet, the model's findings in 1997, that the use of a lamivudine and zidovudine (ZDV) cocktail gives better survival than using ZDV by itself, and that the expenditures for the additional drug give good value for the money spent, have been shown to be true. Thus, the Chancellor model provided valid information on which to base an important clinical policy decision. Since this is the objective of any modeling study, we should consider this a valid model, even though it is would not be an adequate model to use for a study of two HIV drug regimens under consideration for use in 2005.

Discussion

Modeling is a creative endeavor, and at times a risky one. It should always be a multidisciplinary undertaking for several reasons. The model cannot include all clinical trial data, so the most important and valid measures must be selected. This selection process requires the involvement of those who know the clinical trials best: principal investigators, research nurses, monitors, biostatisticians, and others involved in the process. Models also use variables from observational or other databases. These data must be adjusted or analyzed so that the estimates that they bring to the model reflect a level of severity and risk similar to those faced by the trial population. This requires expertise in health services research and epidemiological analysis, and so it is important that clinical trial team members be involved in the modeling process. They should, at a minimum, critique the model design and discuss the value of selecting specific variables and the assumptions that are valid for their data.

No ideal data sources exist to supplement clinical trial data for modeling. It is, therefore, important to cast a broad net to capture several data sources if possible. The use of more than one source of data allows for "triangulation," the identification of several estimates that support each other because they identify a narrow area where the true value may be located.

The identification of a range or cluster of estimates may not seem desirable to some decision makers. There is often a tendency among decision makers to want the "right number," yet finding this elusive value is never possible with a cost-effectiveness modeling study. Indeed, it is not possible for any study involving costs, because true cost is a defined concept not a measurable absolute value. Therefore, in-depth discussion of the strengths and weaknesses of a modeling estimate and of the data and assumptions embodied in this research is required for a good modeling report. In this field, pretension to excessive precision often results in a loss of face validity; it is better to be approximately right than precisely wrong, and a model that does not have face validity is useless for informing critical decisions about how scarce resources are best put to use.

References

1. Simpson KN. Modeling with clinical trial data: Getting from the data researchers have to the data decision makers need. *Drug Information J.* 1995;29:1431–1440.

2. Simpson KN. Problems and perspectives on the use of decision-analysis models for prostate cancer. *J Urol.* 1994;152:1888–1893.

3. Gold M, Siegel J, Russell L, et al., eds. *Cost-Effectiveness in Health and Medicine.* New York: Oxford University Press; 1996.

4. Freedberg KA, Scharfstein JA, Seage GR, et al. The cost-effectiveness of preventing AIDS-related opportunistic infections. *J Am Med Assoc.*1998;279(2):130–136.

5. Simpson KN. Design and assessment of cost effectiveness studies in AIDS populations. *JAIDS.* 1995;10(Suppl.4):S28–S32.

6. Briggs A, Sculpher M. An introduction to Markov modeling for economic evaluation. *Pharmacoeconomics.* 1998;13:397–409.

7. Marshall DA, Simpson KN, Earle CC, Chu CW. Potential cost effectiveness of one-time screening for lung cancer in a high-risk cohort. *Lung Cancer.* 2001;32(3):227–236.

8. Henschke CI, McCauley DI, Yankelevitz DF, et al. Early Lung Cancer Action Project: overall design and findings from baseline screening. *Lancet.* 1999;354(9173):99–105.

9. Sonnenberg FA, Beck JR. Markov models in medical decision making: A practical guide. *Med Decis Making.* 1993;13:322–338.

10. Chancellor JV, Hill AM, Sabin CA, Simpson KN, Youle M. Modeling the cost effectiveness of lamivudine/zidovudine combination therapy in HIV infection. *Pharmacoeconomics.* 1997;12:54–66.

11. Simpson K, Hatziandreu EJ, Andersson F, Shakespeare A, Oleksy I, Tosteson ANA. Cost effectiveness of an antiviral treatment with zalcitabine plus zidovudine for AIDS patients with CD4+ counts less than 300/ml in 5 European countries. *Pharmaco Econ.* 1994;6(6):553–562.

12. Schulman KA, Lynn LA, Glick HA, Eisenberg JM. Cost effectiveness of low-dose zidovudine therapy for asymptomatic patients with human immunodeficiency virus (HIV) infection. *Ann Intern Med.* 1991;114(9):798–802.

13. Freedberg KA, Losina E, Weinstein MC, et al. The cost effectiveness of combination antiretroviral therapy for HIV disease. *N Eng J Med.* 2001;344(11):824–831.

14. Simpson KN, Luo MP, Chumney E, et al. Cost-effectiveness of lopinavir/ritonavir versus nelfinavir as the first-line highly active antiretroviral therapy regimen for HIV infection. *HIV Clinical Trials.* 2004;5(5):294–304.

Section Five

Pharmacoeconomic
Analysis

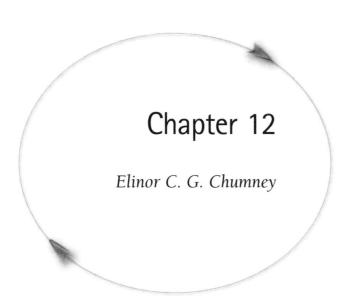

Chapter 12

Elinor C. G. Chumney

Introduction to Pharmacoeconomic Evaluations

The cost of health care has spiraled upwards over the last decade, resulting in increasing calls to somehow limit its growth without jeopardizing the health and well-being of patients throughout the world. This growing emphasis on cost containment has spurred the use of pharmacoeconomic analyses to inform decisions between competing therapies.

The identification of various types of costs and their subsequent measurement in dollars is similar across most economic evaluations; however, the consequences stemming from the alternatives being examined may differ considerably.[1] The simplest form of analysis is the cost minimization analysis (CMA), which compares interventions based on cost alone and directs researchers to choose the lowest cost intervention. In doing so, it assumes that the outcomes (i.e., the benefits or efficacy) of the treatments under consideration are identical.

However, CMA is rarely done, because competing interventions are almost never identically efficacious. In most cases, researchers need a more complex analytic tool to account for different outcomes. In their various forms, pharmacoeconomic evaluations attempt to provide a measure of the benefit derived from a uniform investment of resources. A treatment is considered to be more cost effective than its alternative when it provides a greater benefit for each unit of cost.

Although the United States has made significant progress in its efforts to incorporate cost-effectiveness data into health care decisions at all levels of care, it continues to lag behind other nations. Many providers continue to use cost data instead of formal pharmacoeconomic analysis techniques in determining which drugs to include on formularies. This disparity is particularly apparent when comparisons are made to the way in which other countries, especially those with single-payer systems, incorporate economic evaluation results into their decision-making. Australia and Canada, for example, have recently added cost-effectiveness data to their criteria for health care coverage. In those countries, new treatments must now compete with each other and with existing treatments and must demonstrate greater cost-effectiveness before being included on formularies.

The following chapters are intended as an overview of pharmacoeconomic evaluations. Chapter 14 examines cost-effectiveness analysis (CEA). This is a broad form of pharmacoeconomic analysis in which the numerator measures costs in units of currency and the denominator measures the gain in health in natural units, such as years of life saved or cases of disease averted. Because CEAs can focus on any one of a wide variety of outcome measures, they are limited in both the depth of the information they provide and the generalizability of the results.

The results of a CEA are reported as an incremental cost-effectiveness ratio (ICER) based on the following formula, in which Tx represents "treatment":

$$ICER = \frac{\text{Cost of TxA} - \text{Cost of TxB}}{\text{Effects of TxA} - \text{Effects of TxB}}$$

The lower the ICER, the greater the "bang for the buck" and the more attractive the treatment. Of course, the ICER for a given intervention (TxA) will vary, depending on the comparison treatment (whether TxB or TxC). Although many CEAs compare a new treatment with placebo or with doing nothing, the most *appropriate* comparison treatment is current practice (i.e., the best available treatment). In evaluating studies, it is important to make sure that the relevant strategies are being compared.

Chapter 14 examines cost-utility analysis (CUA). Some consider this to be a special form of either a CEA or cost-benefit analysis (CBA), in which the denominator measures outcomes in quality-adjusted life years (QALYs). Whereas the outcomes in a CEA are unidimensional and program-specific, the outcome measure in a CUA is a composite, allowing for comparisons across programs. There are a number of measurement issues in constructing both utility weights and quality of life measures, and these will be explored in Chapters 15 (Measurement of Utilities) and 16 (Measurement of Health-Related Quality of Life).

Chapter 17 examines CBA, which measures both cost and benefits in units of currency. CBA measures the value of all benefits from an intervention and subtracts from that the measured value of all costs (direct and indirect). Willingness to pay methods typically involve asking contingent valuation questions, thereby allowing respondents to incorporate all dimensions of value into a single dollar amount. In recent years, CBAs have assumed an increasingly important role in pharmacoeconomic and health services research.

Discounting

Regardless of the type of pharmacoeconomic analysis undertaken, researchers must take care to report all costs and benefits in figures that reflect their value in the same baseline year, a process known as discounting. This is an implicit acknowledgement of time preference, the fact that we all value a benefit today more highly than we would value a promise of the same benefit in the future. Very often, treatments result in future benefits as well as a future investment of resources. Although discount rates have varied in the literature and across countries, as long as researchers report the rate they used, their results can be adapted for use with other discount rates. In the United States, 3% is the currently accepted discount rate.[2]

References

1. Drummond MF, O'Brien BJ, Stoddart GL, Torrance GW. Methods for the Economic Evaluation of Health Care Programmes. New York: Oxford University Press, 1997.

2. Gold MR, Siegel JE, Russell LB, Weinstein MC. Cost-effectiveness in Health and Medicine. New York: Oxford University Press, 1996.

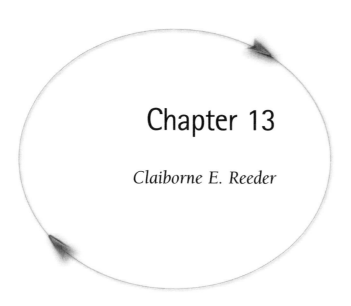

Chapter 13

Claiborne E. Reeder

Cost-Effectiveness Analysis

In a general sense, cost-effectiveness analysis (CEA) is used to evaluate the outcomes and costs of interventions designed to improve health. This technique has been used to compare the economic efficiency of a variety of medical interventions ranging from cancer screening to coronary artery bypass surgery.[1] Information from cost-effectiveness analyses should be used as an *aid* in improving health care decision-making and not as the sole criterion for choice. The ultimate decision to use a particular intervention should incorporate the values of all stakeholders affected by the decision (e.g., providers, payers, and patients). The goal of improving patient outcomes while controlling costs requires data on the clinical, economic, and humanistic costs and consequences of all reasonable therapeutic alternatives available to treat the patient.[2]

Cost-effectiveness analysis is distinguished from cost-benefit analysis (CBA), which will be discussed in a later chapter, in its use of nonmonetary outcome measures. Whereas cost-benefit ratios compare the dollar cost of a treatment with the dollar value of the outcome, cost-effectiveness ratios are calculated as the dollar cost per nonmonetary outcome, such as dollar cost per year of life saved. In other words, a cost-effectiveness ratio (CER) is a measure of the relative *efficiency* of the various treatment alternatives. An efficient treatment is one that achieves the desired outcome or consequence at the lowest cost per outcome. Cost-effectiveness ratios do not provide any information regarding whether or not it is *appropriate* to spend the money to achieve the outcome but rather tell us which treatment provides the lowest cost to achieve the desired outcome. Cost-effectiveness analysis assumes that the funds needed to purchase the most efficient treatment are available. Even when surplus funds are available, cost-effectiveness analyses are still important as they help identify the most efficient use of resources when several treatment options are available. In an era of escalating health care costs, it is critical to include efficiency considerations in our decision-making process.

Two other economic evaluations, cost minimization analysis and cost utility analysis, are actually special cases of the general cost-effectiveness technique; these pharmacoeconomic methods are discussed separately in other chapters.

In terms of pharmaceuticals, cost-effectiveness analysis is used to compare the cost and consequences (outcomes) of two or more treatment alternatives in achieving a particular therapeutic objective.[3-5] For example, a recent study evaluated the cost-effectiveness threshold of ciprofloxacin 0.3% and dexamethasone 0.1% otic suspension relative to ofloxacin otic solution for the treatment of acute otis media in pediatric patients with tympanostomy tubes.[6]

In a cost-effectiveness analysis, the consequences or outcomes of the treatment alternatives are measured in the same nonmonetary units, such as life-years saved, percentage reduction in lipid levels or, as in the example above, cases cured. Results from different cost-effectiveness analyses can be compared as long as the alternatives are specified with the same outcome measure. For example, the effects of diet and exercise on blood pressure can be compared with an antihypertensive medication regimen as long as the outcomes of both treatments are measured on the same metric, such as systolic blood pressure or risk of stroke. In a cost-effectiveness analysis, the outcome measure used should relate to the "true" consequence of interest.[7] For example, in a cost-effectiveness study of persons with type II diabetics, HbA_1C levels could be used to measure a drug's efficacy. In reality, we are not interested in the HbA_1C levels per se, but rather how well these levels correlate with the undesired consequences of diabetes such as diabetic neuropathy and vision loss. If controlling HbA_1C level reduces the long-term consequences of type II diabetes, this lab value can be used as a surrogate for treatment outcome.

Design and Conduct of Cost–Effectiveness Studies

The basics for conducting cost-effectiveness analyses have been outlined by Warner and Luce and summarized nicely by Bootman et al.[4,5] into six general steps.

1—Define the Problem

The first step in conducting a cost-effectiveness analysis should be identification of the research problem. Appropriate literature should be reviewed to support the nature and scope of the problem. For example, there are several medications (e.g., aspirin, streptokinase, and tissue plasminogen activator [tPA]) used in the treatment of patients with an acute myocardial infarction (AMI). Each of these medications varies in costs and effectiveness, so the question of relative efficiency in treating an AMI is a clinically and economically important problem. In addition to identifying the problem, the goal and specific objectives of the study should also be stated clearly in the problem step. For example, is the aim of the study to compare all treatment options or only those admini-stered directly in the emergency department? Will the study include all MI patients or just those within specific age groups? Last, the problem identification step should state the *perspective* of the study. The perspective of a study refers to the intended audience; that is, the individuals or organizations that will use the results of the study in their decision-making process. The study perspective is important because it will influence which costs and outcomes will be included in the study and how they will be quantified. The study perspective may be broad and encompassing or narrow and focused. The *societal perspective* is the broadest and would include all costs and benefits regardless of who pays for the treatment and who benefits. A societal perspective has been recommended by the Panel on Cost-Effectiveness in Health and Medicine as the one that should be used in health policy decisions that would affect the public.[1] However, in practice, most pharmaco-economic evaluations are conducted from a particular perspective such as a hospital, managed care organization, payer, or employer viewpoint. When a particular perspective is specified, only the cost and outcomes relevant to that perspective are included in the analysis, while others are omitted. For example, a study to evaluate which of several lipid-lowering agents is most cost effective for a state Medicaid program formulary should include all the costs for which the Medicaid program would provide benefits relative to lipid reduction treatment as well as all the benefits that accrue to Medicaid for making the drug readily available (such as a reduced rate of cardiovascular disease and decreased medical costs). Because Medicaid is a public program that pays for most of the medical care for people in the program, the broader, societal perspective is appropriate. In contrast, a private health plan (insurer) might only be interested in the costs it will pay directly and the benefits it will realize directly from paying for the treatment.

2—Identify Relevant Treatment Alternatives

The problem statement frames which alternatives should be compared in a cost-effectiveness analysis. A cost-effectiveness analysis will always compare two or more alternative treatments; occasionally one of the alternatives may be "do nothing," provide supportive care, or use a placebo. A useful cost-effectiveness analysis will compare treatment alternatives that are currently used in practice with the newer therapy. This type of comparison is often referred to as a "head-to-head" or "active control" trial.

Whether a treatment alternative is relevant or not should be a function of the problem statement and study perspective. For example, suppose we are interested in reducing hypertension in a working population of people between the ages of 25 and 55 years. In this case, we might include diet and exercise as well as drug therapy to decrease blood pressure. In another situation, we might be interested in the most efficient way to treat hypertension in elderly patients who are also diabetic. In this case our treatment alternatives might be limited to an evaluation of agents within a particular therapeutic class, such as ACE inhibitors and diuretics, that may be available as part of a senior drug benefit program.

3—Describe the Relationship Between Resource Inputs and Outcomes

Once the problem has been stated clearly and relevant alternatives specified, the next step is to describe the relationship between resource inputs and outcomes. Economists refer to this relationship as the "production process" for treatment; clinicians might describe the production process in terms of a clinical pathway or treatment algorithm. In a production process, resource inputs are those products and services needed to produce a given outcome or output. Examples of inputs to medical care production include medications, physician visits, hospitalizations, laboratory tests, and nursing care. These inputs are brought together in the production process, where outcomes are produced. The "production" takes place in a variety of settings, such as the physician's office, ambulatory clinic, hospital, emergency department, pharmacy, or the patient's home. Outcomes are can be categorized as either resource outcomes or health outcomes. Resource outcomes reflect the changes in resource use, such as medications and physician visits, that can be attributed to the intervention. Health outcomes reflect the impact of the intervention on patient biomedical functioning (e.g., blood pressure, cardiac output), mortality, morbidity, and humanistic outcomes (e.g., patient satisfaction and health-related quality of life). Figure 13-1 depicts the concept of a health care production process.

A useful technique to illustrate the clinical relationship between resource inputs and outcomes is a decision tree. A decision tree (Figure 13-2) can be used to represent or model the clinical decision-

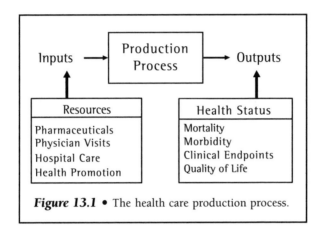

Figure 13.1 • The health care production process.

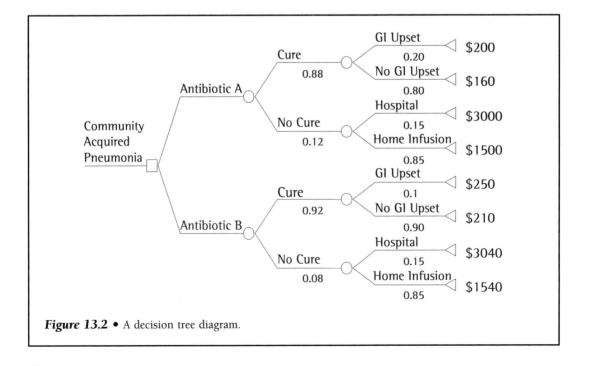

Figure 13.2 • A decision tree diagram.

making process and related outcomes. The decision tree depicts the clinical production process for the analysis; inputs are ordered chronologically from left to right and lead to the possible outcomes (outputs) of treatment. These outcomes may be desired outcomes (increased survival) or unintended outcomes (adverse drug events). For more information on decision trees, see Chapter 5.

Establishing evidence of efficacy and effectiveness is critical to conducting a valid pharmaco-economic evaluation. Evidence of efficacy and effectiveness can be garnered from a variety of sources, which can vary in the strength and quality of the evidence that they provide. The most common sources of efficacy and effectiveness data for pharmacoeconomic studies are clinical trials, effectiveness trials, meta analyses, observational studies, and database studies. The strength of the evidence is a function of how well the study was designed and conducted. Randomized controlled trials with large numbers of subjects provide the strongest scientific evidence of efficacy, while small observational studies provide the weakest level of evidence.

The distinction between efficacy and effectiveness is important in understanding how much the results of an economic evaluation may be generalized. *Efficacy* measures the effect of a medical treatment (drug, procedure, device) under well-controlled scientific conditions, such as in randomized controlled trials (RCTs). RCTs provide evidence that the intervention can work, at least under certain circumstances. In the past, adoption of a new drug therapy was based largely on the results of randomized controlled trials that showed that the drug was safe and efficacious relative to placebo. Little, if any, consideration was given to the cost of the drug. As the cost of health care in general and pharmaceuticals in particular increased, emphasis shifted from just an emphasis on efficacy to inclusion of effectiveness and cost.

Effectiveness measures the outcomes of drugs and other medical interventions under real-world practice conditions. Effectiveness differs from efficacy because in the daily use of medicines, physicians prescribe and patients use the medicines much differently than how they were used in the clinical trial protocols. Factors such as compliance, age, ethnicity, genetics, and comorbidity influence patient response to treatment. Consequently the effectiveness of a new medicine is typically less than its efficacy.

When costs are considered along with efficacy and effectiveness, the question of efficiency arises. *Efficiency* deals with how well resources are used in producing health care outcomes. In pharmaco-economic terms, a new drug or treatment would be the most efficient if it delivered the desired outcome for the lowest possible cost. In this sense, pharmacoeconomic ratios can be thought of as efficiency ratios.

Cost-effectiveness studies use data from both efficacy and effectiveness trials to estimate efficiency. When a study uses the results of randomized controlled trials to estimate efficiency, the study is a cost efficacy analysis and represents the efficiency of the intervention under the ideal conditions of the trial. When these data are obtained from effectiveness trials, the efficiency estimate (pharmacoeconomic ratio) is more likely to mirror what will be seen in the real world and represents the cost-effectiveness of the drug.

Meta analysis has become a popular source of efficacy and effectiveness data for pharmacoeconomic analyses. Meta analysis is a systematic approach to identifying and integrating the results of a number of clinical trials into a meaningful summary. Through "pooling" efficacy data from similar clinical trials, meta analyses may provide estimates of the efficacy of interventions that are more precise than those reported in the individual trials.

Health care databases are another useful source of effectiveness data. Paid claims databases from private insurers, health care plans, and employers provide a rich source of information on utilization and cost of treatment in the daily practice of medicine (i.e., effectiveness). While not as scientifically rigorous as randomized controlled trials, database analyses employ epidemiological and statistical methods as well as large numbers of patient records to provide reasonably valid and reliable estimates of effectiveness and treatment outcomes.

Results from clinical trials, effectiveness studies, and meta analyses are used to determine the probabilities of events and outcomes in economic studies. These data are used to populate decision tree models that are then used to estimate average treatment cost.

4—Identify Cost and Outcomes of Treatment Alternatives

Once the clinical treatment pathway (decision tree) is specified, resource costs and outcomes for each alternative can be incorporated. Identifying relevant costs and consequences associated with the use of pharmaceutical products and services are important tasks in any pharmacoeconomic evaluation. Deciding which cost and consequences to include in a pharmacoeconomic study and how to value them is a function of the study perspective. The broadest perspective is *societal* and would include the full range of cost and consequences listed in Table 13-1. If the study is conducted from a narrower perspective, such as a payer or provider perspective, cost and consequences in the indirect and intangible categories may not be included in the analysis. In contrast, a study conducted from an employer or patient perspective might include the effects of treatment on productivity and quality of life. It is important to understand the study perspective and to evaluate the appropriateness of the perspective. A good pharmacoeconomic study will always state and justify the perspective used in the analysis.

Costs and consequences (outcomes) may be classified into three major groups: direct, indirect, and intangible.[4,8] Table 13-1 provides some frequently encountered examples of these types of costs and outcomes.

Direct costs include both medical and nonmedical expenditure for the detection, treatment, and prevention of disease. *Direct medical costs* reflect resources consumed in the "production" of medical care such as pharmaceutical products and services, physician visits, laboratory monitoring, and hospital care. *Direct nonmedical costs* reflect expenditures for products and services that are not directly related to disease treatment, but are still proximately related to patient care. Examples of direct nonmedical costs include transportation cost to a pharmacy or physician's office and caregiver costs

Table 13.1
Examples of Resource Costs and Consequences

Direct Medical	Indirect
• Physician office visits	• Lost productivity due to death or illness
• Hospital care	• Absenteeism
• Pharmaceutical products and services	• Changes in productivity due to morbidity
• Outpatient medical care	
• Laboratory tests	Intangible
• Diagnostic tests and procedures	• Changes in health-related quality of life
	• Social and emotional well-being
Direct Nonmedical	• Life satisfaction
• Transportation costs to obtain care	
• Housekeeping costs	
• Custodial care for dependents	

during the illness period. Frequently, direct nonmedical costs are paid out-of-pocket by the patient or assumed as an unreimbursed cost of care.

Indirect costs account for changes in productivity of an individual because illness leads to absenteeism and "presenteeism." Absenteeism reflects the time a person is actually away from the job, while presenteeism reflects the decrease in productivity when working ill. The monetary value of lost or altered productivity is typically used as a measure of indirect costs. Two approaches used to estimate productivity costs are the "human capital" approach and the "willingness-to-pay" approach. The human capital approach estimates productivity changes based on the average wages for individuals in the work force.[7]

The willingness-to-pay method measures productivity costs as the value individuals attribute to health and well-being or to avoiding symptoms of disease. Economists typically prefer the willingness-to-pay approach because it considers a variety of costs that may not be included in the human capital approach. Conceptually, willingness-to-pay captures not only lost wages, but also the value individuals place on humanistic outcomes such as pain avoidance and social functioning. Unfortunately use of the willingness-to-pay approach to estimate indirect costs is limited by several factors, such as the ability of individuals to accurately judge value under hypothetical situations and the variability of risk-taking behavior among individuals.

Intangible costs and consequences are nonmonetary in nature and reflect the impact of a disease and its treatment on the social and emotional functioning of individuals and their quality of life. These humanistic consequences are measured using health-related quality of life instruments and patient satisfaction questionnaires. Humanistic outcomes are also known as Patient Reported Outcomes (PROs). Examples of such instruments are discussed in another chapter.

When costs and consequences occur over an extended period of time (usually more than one year) then these amounts need to be adjusted to reflect the "time value of money." To accurately compare the costs and benefits of a medical intervention, both must be related to the same point in time. The time value of money recognizes the influence of inflation and interest rates on monetary worth. In simple terms, a dollar today is worth more than a dollar received in the future. For example, if you have a choice between receiving a payment of $100 today or the same $100 payment a year from now, it is financially preferable to take the money now because of interest rates and inflation.

The technique used to account for the time value of money is called "discounting." In discounting, the net present value of future cash inflows or outflows is calculated. Adjusting the value of future costs and consequences to account for inflation and interest portrays these amounts in today's dollars. For example, if interest rates were 4% per year, you could actually accept a payment of $96.15 today in lieu of a $100 payment a year from now and be just as well off financially. Why? Because the $96.15 could be invested at 4% interest for the year and be worth $100 at the end of the year ($96.15 + (96.15)(0.04) = $100). The $96.15 is referred to as the "net present value" of $100 received one year from now. Discounting future costs and benefits recognizes the time value of money.

For example, two vaccines, X and Y, can be used for prevention of "epizuditis." Vaccine X is expected to save $10,000 per year in medical costs over the next 3 years for a total savings of $30,000. Vaccine Y is also expected to save a total of $30,000 in medical costs over the next 3 years, but the flow of savings is different for Drug Y. Drug Y would save $20,000 in the first year and $5,000 in each of the second and third years. While both vaccines save a total of $30,000 in medical costs, we would prefer to use Drug Y because a larger portion of the savings accrue in the first year and the discounted value of the savings for Drug Y would be higher than for Drug X. For a more detailed discussion of discounting, see Bootman et al.[4] Discounting is very important when costs and benefits of treatments accrue unevenly over time (as in the vaccine example), when inflation and interest rates are high, or when the time period for the comparison is longer than 1 year.

5—Valuing Resource Cost and Outcomes

Once all relevant costs and consequences for a treatment pathway have been identified, the value (cost) of each item must be determined. Resource and outcome costing has two components: the quantity of resources consumed and the price of each unit of resource.[3] The quantity of resources is measured as the amount of resources used in the care (production) process. The price of the resource should reflect the amount actually paid, (i.e., the cost) to purchase the resource or input.

There are several methods for measuring and determining resource use and costs in an economic study. First, resource use and costs can be collected concurrently as part of a clinical trial protocol. With this approach, the quantities of resources used in treatment are collected along side the clinical data. When economic data are collected as part of a clinical trial, there may be resources consumed that would not be used in routine daily practice. These are known as protocol-induced costs. When economic data are not collected as part of the clinical trial, resource use may be determined by examining patient charts or databases. Second, resource use may be determined by patient or provider interviews. Patient diaries are frequently used to track the types and quantities of resources consumed by patients during their course of treatment. Health care providers, such a physicians, pharmacists, and nurses, can also provide information on the resources used and the outcomes of treatment. Third, administrative databases can be used to extract utilization and cost data. Health plans maintain claims files for all services paid for by the plan. To the extent that these files contain diagnosis and procedure codes, they can be used to determine resource use patterns for the treatment of specific diseases.

Once the quantity of resources is determined, a relevant price must be attached to each unit of the resource that is consumed. For example, if a hospitalized patient receives two vials of an IV antibiotic per day for 5 days, the total consumption is 10 vials. Next, a price must be determined for each vial. The relevant price that is used is a function of the study perspective. If the study were being done from the provider (hospital) perspective, the price would be that actually paid for the drug by the hospital. If this were $120 per vial, the resource cost for this drug would be $1200. If the study were done from a payer perspective, such as the health plan or patient, the relevant price would be the amount actually paid by the plan or patient. So if the hospital charged the patient $200 per vial, the relevant price of the drug from the patient's perspective would be $2000. As shown by this illustration, the decision to use cost or charges in an economic evaluation should be determined by the perspective of the study.

There are basically two approaches to assigning a price to resource use: market price and reference price. Market price reflects the amount actually paid by the producer to acquire the resource. In the example above, this would be $120 per vial of antibiotic. The second approach, a reference price, is used when actual market prices are unknown and must be estimated. Reference prices are obtained from external sources and reflect prices that are available in the general market place. A commonly used reference price for pharmaceuticals is the Average Wholesale Price (AWP), which is a readily available, standard price in the public domain. When studies use data from administrative claims, it is often difficult to determine the actual cost of resource as these databases typically contain charge data, which may not reflect the actual amounts, paid. In these cases, reference prices may be used to reflect a more realistic estimate of the real price.

6—Interpretation and Presentation of Results

Once all cost and consequences have been measured and the effectiveness of the treatment alternatives is determined, the relative cost-effectiveness of the treatments can be estimated. This is done by ranking the treatments in order of their cost and effectiveness and eliminating those options, which are most costly and more expensive (i.e., dominated). Next, the ratios can be calculated and ranked to determine which of the alternatives is most efficient.

The idea of relative cost-effectiveness and dominance is illustrated in Figure 13-3. A treatment may be considered cost-effective in three cases: (1) when it is more effective and less costly than the others, (2) when it is more effective and more expensive, but adds value, and (3) when it less effective and less expensive.(3) Dominant alternatives are those that are more effective and less expensive than other treatments (case 1). In cases 2 and 3, trade-offs are made regarding whether the increase (decrease) in cost is worth the increase (decrease) in effectiveness.

Before making any conclusions from a pharmacoeconomic study, however, it is important to understand the limitations of the study and how the results relate to a particular practice setting. In a simple cost-effectiveness analysis, the results may be presented as a single, *average* cost-effectiveness ratio, such as $28,000 per year of life saved. To be meaningful, this ratio should be presented in comparison to other treatment alternatives, preferably the current standard of practice or treatment. When presented as the only measure of efficiency, average cost-effectiveness ratios can be misleading. It is important to remember that these numbers are *ratios* and, thus, contain a numerator and a denominator. The numerator and denominator should be evaluated to assure that the cost and effects of the treatment are meaningful to the treatment decision. For example, if we were asked to name the most cost-effective drug to lower lipid levels, a logical choice, based on cost-effectiveness ratios, would be generic niacin tablets. Why? Because it works (lowers lipid levels by 5%–10%), and it is cheap (pennies per tablet). Niacin would have a very favorable *average* CER, but few would argue that it would be the drug of choice for patients who need a substantial reduction in lipid levels. A classic example of how average CE ratios can be misleading is illustrated in an article in the *New England Journal of Medicine* in 1975.[12] The article compared the average CERs with the incremental CERs for conducting consecutive screening tests for blood in the stool (a marker for colon cancer). The average cost-effectiveness ratio for conducting six consecutive tests was $2,451 per case detected, while the incremental cost-effectiveness ratio for the sixth test was $47,107,214 per additional case detected.

		Cost of A Versus B		
		Lower	Equal	Higher
Effectiveness of A Versus B	Higher	Choose A Dominant	Choose A	Trade-off
	Equal	Choose A	Equality	Choose B
	Lower	Trade-off	Choose B	Choose B Dominant

Figure 13.3 • A cost-effectiveness grid and the concept of dominance.
Source: References 3 and 4.

While the average CER per case detected seems reasonable, the incremental ratio for the sixth test was astronomical. This disparity in the average and incremental ratios existed because most of the benefit of screening resulted from the first of the six tests; the additional benefit of the other tests was very small, but the costs were substantial.

Average and incremental cost-effectiveness ratios are often presented in the form of *league tables, which* rank treatments according to their cost-effectiveness ratios and serves to guide decisions of which treatment is most efficient. While league tables are a convenient method of presenting cost-effectiveness ratios, there is some disagreement on their usefulness in decision-making. Differences in study designs, treatment populations, and study time may make meaningful comparisons difficult.

A more informative measure to assess the relative value of alternative treatments is the incremental cost-effectiveness ratio. The incremental cost-effectiveness ratio compares the relative change in effectiveness of two treatments to the relative change in cost. It is calculated by dividing the difference in costs of two treatments by the difference in effectiveness of the two treatments. Presentation of the incremental cost-effectiveness ratio is very important when one treatment is both more effective and more costly than the treatment alternative. Another method for illustrating the incremental cost-effectiveness of one treatment versus another is the cost-effectiveness plane (Figure 13-4). The cost-effectiveness plane depicts the incremental cost of the two treatments on the Y axis and the incremental effectiveness on the X axis.[4,13] The four quadrants of the cost-effectiveness plane parallel those of the cost-effectiveness grid in Figure 13-3. In Quadrant I, treatment A is more effective and more costly than B and, thus, requires a determination of whether the added benefit is worth the added cost. In Quadrant II, treatment A is dominant as it is both more effective and less costly than B. If treatment A is both less costly and less effective than B (Quadrant III), a trade-off decision is needed. That is, is it clinically reasonable to accept some reduction in effectiveness for a significant reduction in cost? Finally, if treatment A is both more costly and less effective than B, treatment B will dominate the use of A.

When interpreting the results of a study, one should pay particular attention to the estimates used for resource utilization and costs. Assumptions are made in all pharmacoeconomic analyses regarding the likelihood (probability) of occurrence of desired or undesired effects, the cost or value of inputs and outcomes, and the perspective of the analysis. With assumptions come uncertainties in results. Sensitivity analysis addresses this uncertainty by varying model assumptions over some reasonable and relevant range of values to investigate whether the results would change. The more stable the results are over this relevant range of the values, the more confidence we can have in the results. Studies in which the results do not change significantly when assumptions are relaxed are said to be "robust."

What constitutes a relevant range of values over which the robustness should be tested? This question can best be answered from a clinical standpoint. What change would a clinician believe to be meaningful? For example, if compliance with a new asthma drug was reported in the clinical trials to be 95%, it is unlikely that we will observe a higher compliance rate in the actual practice. We would be more interested in the effects of lower compliance rates of perhaps 60%–70% on patient outcomes. If the drug is still effective when compliance decreases from 95% to 70%, we could be reasonably confident that LowTack will perform well in actual practice. As a general rule, sensitivity analyses should be conducted on all important study variables and should include a range of values that are clinically believable.

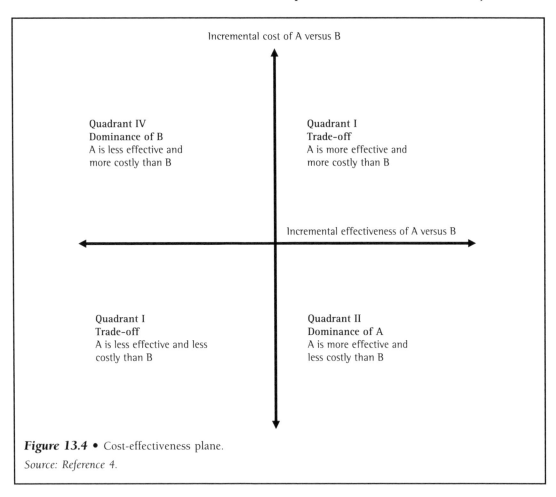

Figure 13.4 • Cost-effectiveness plane.
Source: Reference 4.

Cost–Effectiveness Analysis: Example

A new inhaled therapy for the management of acute attacks of asthma has been tested in a randomized controlled clinical trial. In the trial, the new therapy (LowTack) was compared to the current standard of treatment (EZBreathe). The outcome of interest in the trial was symptom-free days, a nonmonetary measure. Economic data were captured as part of the clinical trial, because the company thought their product might offer not only a clinical advantage but also an economic advantage. Given the nonmonetary outcome of symptom-free days, a cost-effectiveness analysis was conducted. The study was conducted from a third-party payer perspective, and only direct medical costs (drug costs, physician office visits, emergency department visits) were included in the analysis, and market prices were used to determine resource unit costs. The number of days without any breathing problems (symptom-free days) was recorded by the patient over a 3-month period in a diary. Medical resource utilization was abstracted from patient charts and study records. The average total cost of treatment per patient and the average number of symptom-free days per patient for each drug are summarized in Table 13-2.

Table 13.2
Average Treatment Costs and Outcomes

Drug	Average Treatment Cost Per Month	Symptom-free Days Per Month
LowTack	$ 43.20	24
EZBreathe	$ 32.00	20

Average Cost-Effectiveness Ratios

The average cost-effectiveness ratio is calculated for each treatment by dividing the treatment cost by the number of symptom-free days for each drug.

For LowTack:

$C/E_{LowTack} = (Cost_{LowTack}) / (Symptom\text{-}free\ days_{LowTack})$

$C/E_{LowTack} = \$43.20 / 24\ days$

$C/E_{LowTack} = \$1.80$ per symptom-free day

For EZBreathe:

$C/E_{EZBreathe} = (Cost_{EZBreathe}) / (Symptom\text{-}free\ days_{EZBreathe})$

$C/E_{EZBreathe} = \$32.00 / 20\ days$

$C/E_{EZBreathe} = \$1.60$ per symptom-free day

Based on these average cost-effectiveness ratios, EZBreathe, the current standard of treatment is the most cost-effective agent (lowest cost per outcome).

The average cost-effectiveness ratio reflects the cost to achieve an outcome (symptom-free day) independent of other treatments. If this were all the information available, EZBreathe would be the choice. However, while LowTack costs more than EZBreathe, it is also more efficacious (more symptom-free days). LowTack would be located in Quadrant I of Figure 13-4; it is more effective than EZBreathe and also more costly. The cost-effectiveness ratio is simply a measure of efficiency and does not tell us whether or not it is appropriate to spend more money for greater efficacy. A more informed choice can be made by looking at the incremental cost-effectiveness ratio, which tells us how much we would have to pay to achieve the additional efficacy of LowTack over EZBreathe.[10]

Incremental Cost-Effectiveness Ratio

When one treatment is both more effective and more expensive than another, the real question is how much it costs to receive the additional or incremental benefit. The incremental cost-effectiveness ratio (ICER) is calculated by dividing the incremental change in cost of two therapies by the incremental change in effectiveness.[10]

$ICER_{LowTack\ vs\ EZBreathe} = (Cost_{LowTack} - Cost_{EZBreathe}) / (Symptom\text{-}free\ days_{LowTack} - Symptom\text{-}free\ days_{EZBreathe})$

$ICER = (\$43.20 - \$32.00) / (24\ days - 20\ days)$

ICER = ($11.20 / 4 days)

ICER = $2.80 for each additional symptom-free day

The decision is now one of clinical and economic judgment, and not mathematics: Is it worth $2.80 to achieve an additional day free of asthma symptoms? In this case, it might be easy to agree. In other cases, it will be much more difficult to decide.

For example, two treatments (A and B) both improve survival: Treatment A by 22 years and Treatment B by 22.5 years. The average cost-effectiveness ratios are $15,000 per year of life saved for A and $16,000 per year of life saved for B. Based on these ratios, it might be tempting to pay an additional $1,000 *on average* more for Treatment B. However, the incremental cost-effectiveness ratio shows that an additional year of life saved would cost $60,000, not the $1,000 difference in average cost of the two drugs. Unfortunately, there are no generally accepted amounts or ranges to judge when an intervention is acceptable in terms of its cost-effectiveness.

Incremental cost-effectiveness ratios are the preferred measure of relative value because they allow the decision maker to see the cost of the additional benefit of one treatment compared to another. Whether the additional expenditure is appropriate is a matter of choice and should include clinical, economic and humanistic considerations.[11]

Sensitivity Analysis

The purpose of a sensitivity analysis is to assess how much the results of a study might change if certain assumptions about utilization and cost were varied. As the cost of medical care (drugs, physician visits, ED visits, hospital cost) increase each year and certainly vary among suppliers and regions of the country, it is important to account for such potential differences when estimating cost-effectiveness. In addition to variations in costs, assumptions about effectiveness should also be varied, as they too can influence the results. In this case, we would probably like to know the effects of a 30% increase in drug price or the effects of emergency department use being 10% greater than anticipated. A good cost-effectiveness analysis will make all assumptions clear and will include a sensitivity analysis to assess the effects of variations in key cost and utilization drivers. A sensitivity analysis would recalculate the CE ratios with the higher price to answer this question.

To illustrate, suppose in this example that the cost of LowTack increased by $6 per month or $0.25 per day. Would this increase in drug cost alter our results and conclusions? The effect of this change is to increase the average cost per symptom-free day from $1.80 to $2.05 and the incremental cost-effectiveness ratio from $2.80 per additional symptom-free day to $4.30. The decision is still one of balancing the gain in effectiveness with the increase in cost. In general, sensitivity analyses will vary important utilization and cost parameters over a reasonable range of values to show the strength of robustness of the model and help us make more informed decisions.

Summary

Cost-effectiveness analysis is a type of pharmacoeconomic technique that can be used to compare the cost and outcomes of two of more treatments when the outcomes are measured in the same nonmonetary unit. An average cost-effectiveness ratio is a measure of the efficiency of a treatment in that it indicates the average cost to achieve a desired outcome. Cost-effectiveness ratios for treatments with the same outcome measure can be compared to determine which is most efficient. Average cost-effectiveness ratios indicate the efficiency of an intervention independent of other available treatments. Used in isolation, average cost-effectiveness ratios can be somewhat misleading because they only measure efficiency relative to other treatment options. Incremental cost-effectiveness ratios present the incremental change in cost relative to the incremental change in outcomes and, thus, provide a measure of relative efficiency. Incremental cost-effectiveness ratios are more appropriate measures when making therapy choices. When the results of a cost-effectiveness analysis are presented, they should present study limitations and assumptions in a very transparent manner. Sensitivity analyses should be conducted for all key assumptions in the analysis so that the reader can appreciate how robust the results are to variations that are likely to occur in real world practice.

Pharmacoeconomic ratios provide us with another tool to improve our treatment decisions. These tools should not be used in isolation from other factors in the treatment process. Rather than telling us which drug to use, pharmacoeconomic ratios inform us about the circumstances under which a treatment is most efficient. Incorporating efficiency criteria in our decision-making is necessary and desirable given the escalating demand for newer, more expensive treatments and the constant pressure to control health care costs.

References

1. Gold MR, Siegel JE, Russell LB, Weinstein MC. *Cost-Effectiveness in Health and Medicine*. New York: Oxford University Press; 1996.
2. Kozma CM, Reeder CE, Schulz RM. Economic, clinical, and humanistic outcomes: a planning model for pharmacoeconomic research. *Clin Ther.* 1993;15(6).
3. Drummond MF, O'Brien B, Stoddart GL, Torrance GW. *Methods for the Economic Evaluation of Healthcare Programmes*. Oxford: Oxford University Press, 1977.
4. Bootman JL. Townsend RJ, McGhan WF. *Principles of Pharmacoeconomics*. Cincinnati, OH: Harvey Whitney Books Company, 2005.
5. Warner KE, Luce BR. *Cost-Benefit and Cost-Effectiveness Analysis and Health Care: Principles Practice and Potential*. Ann Arbor, MI: Health Administration Press, 1982.
6. Roland PS, Pontius A, Wall GM, Waycaster CR. A cost threshold analysis of ciprofloxacin-dexamethasone versus ofloxacin for acute otitis media in pediatric patients with tympanostomy tubes. *Clin Ther.* 2004;26(7):1168–1178.
7. Berger ML, Bingefors K, Hedblom EC, et al. *Health Care Cost, Quality, and Outcomes: ISPOR Book of Terms*. International Society for Pharmacoeconomics and Outcomes Research; 2003.
8. Eisenberg JM. Clinical economics: a guide to the economic analysis of clinical practices. *JAMA.* 1989; 262:2879–2886.
9. Luce BR, Elixhauser A. *Standards for Socioeconomic Evaluation of Health Care Products and Services*. Germany: Springer-Verlag; 1990.
10. Kielhorn A, Graf von der Schulenburg J-M. *The Health Economics Handbook*. Paris: Adis; 2000.
11. Kozma CM. Consideration of cost-consequence ratios as an emerging tool in pharmacoeconomic decision making. *New Med.* 1997;1:35–39.
12. Neuhauser D, Lewicki AM. What do we gain from the sixth stool guaiac? *N Engl J Med.* 1975;293:226–228.
13. Black WC. The CE plane: a graphical representation of cost-effectiveness. *Med Decision Making.* 1990; 10:212–214.

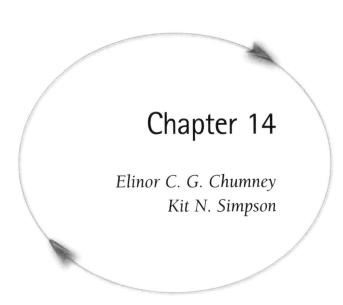

Chapter 14

Elinor C. G. Chumney
Kit N. Simpson

Cost-Utility Analysis

Recall from Chapter 13 that in a cost-effectiveness analysis (CEA), the incremental cost of a program is compared with the incremental health effects of that program, and the health effects are measured in natural units such as life-years gained. Although widely used and important in its own right, there are two main drawbacks with this form of analysis. The first is that a CEA focuses on a single outcome of effect even though a given medical intervention may actually have a spectrum of outcomes of interest. These could include life-years gained, physiologic improvements or compromises, treatment side effects, and other quality-of-life issues. A second and related limitation is that the resulting incremental cost-effectiveness ratios (ICERs) cannot be compared when different units of health effects have been used for different programs.

To overcome these problems with a traditional CEA, researchers often turn to a cost-utility analysis (CUA). It is frequently treated as simply a special form of CEA in which the denominator is standardized to measure outcomes in quality-adjusted life years (QALYs).[1,2] The construction of QALYs recognizes that the output of a particular health care intervention cannot be considered merely in terms of extra years of life; it adjusts or weights the resulting years of life by the quality of those years. This adjustment accounts for the fact that there are two important aspects of any intervention: (1) the resulting quantity of life (life expectancy or mortality) and (2) the resulting quality of life (morbidity, which is more difficult to measure). As a uniform measure of health outcome, the QALY is designed to simultaneously reflect gains from the reduction of both morbidity and mortality resulting from a given intervention.[1]

The results of a CUA are presented in an ICER ($/QALY), alternatively known as an incremental cost-utility ratio (ICUR). This ratio indicates the cost required to generate the equivalent of one additional year of perfect health (1 QALY).

By providing a method through which these various outcomes can be combined into a single composite outcome (the QALY), CUA allows researchers to compare their results with those of other CUA studies. In so doing, it greatly facilitates interdisease as well as intradisease comparisons; magnetic resonance imaging (MRI) scans can then be compared with both Doppler screening and aspirin therapy to determine which program generates the greatest utility for a given monetary investment (see Table 14.1).

CUA is most appropriately used in the following situations[1]:

1. When health-related quality of life is the important outcome.

   For example, researchers comparing alternative treatments for arthritis evaluate the programs based on how well they improve the patients' physical, social, and psychological functioning; arthritis treatments are not expected to have an effect on patient mortality.

2. When health-related quality of life is one of the important outcomes (i.e., when the program affects both morbidity and mortality).

   For example, many cancer treatments improve both longevity and long-term quality of life but can significantly decrease the patients' quality of life in the short term (during the treatment process itself).

3. When the programs being compared have a wide range of different outcomes.

   For example, decision makers wanting to maximize the health benefits with a limited budget must have a common tool to evaluate the expected health benefits derived from a uniform investment of resources in competing programs.

4. When researchers wish to compare a program to others that have already been evaluated using a CUA.

   For example, a formulary committee deciding whether or not to expand its list to include the latest drugs for a number of different conditions must have a common tool to evaluate the expected health benefits.

As mentioned earlier in Chapter 13, health care providers around the world are increasingly using cost-effectiveness data to determine which pharmaceuticals to cover in drug formularies. Other nations, such as Australia and Canada, have recently added cost-effectiveness data to their criteria for

Table 14.1
League Table of CUAs with Ratios Converted to 1998 U.S. Dollars

Intervention	Comparator	Target Population	Reference	$/QALY
Warfarin	Aspirin	65-year-old with nonvalvular atrial fibrillation and high risk for stroke	Gage et al. (1995)[3]	Cost-saving
Warfarin	Aspirin	65-year-old with nonvalvular atrial fibrillation and medium risk for stroke	Gage et al. (1995)[3]	Cost-saving
Fortification with folic acid at 0.7 mg/100 g cereal grain product	No fortification program to prevent congenital abnormalities	All women in U.S. capable of becoming pregnant	Gold et al. (1996)[2]	Cost-saving
Pneumococcal pneumonia vaccination	No vaccination	People >64 years old	Sisk et al. (1997)[4]	Cost-saving
Nefazodone	Step approach (nefazodone if imipramine fails)	30-year-old women with one previous episode of major depression	Revicki et al. (1997)[5]	$2,800
Captopril	No captopril	80-year-old patients surviving myocardial infarction	Tsevat et al. (1995)[6]	$4,300
Nefazodone	Imipramine	30-year-old women with one previous episode of major depression	Revicki et al. (1997)[5]	$4,500
Captopril	No captopril	70-year-old patients surviving myocardial infarction	Tsevat et al. (1995)[6]	$5,900
Fluoxetine	Imipramine	30-year-old women with one previous episode of major depression	Revicki et al. (1997)[5]	$7,000
Warfarin	Aspirin	65-year-old with nonvalvular atrial fibrillation and medium risk for stroke	Gage et al. (1995)[3]	$8,800
Warfarin	No therapy	65-year-old with nonvalvular atrial fibrillation and low risk for stroke	Gage et al. (1995)[3]	$15,000
Interferon-α2b with melphalan and prednisone	Conventional treatment	Patients with multiple myeloma	Nord et al. (1997)[7]	$19,000

(continued)

Table 14.1 (cont'd)
League Table of CUAs with Ratios Converted to 1998 U.S. Dollars

Intervention	Comparator	Target Population	Reference	$/QALY
Driver-side air bag	No air bags	Driving population and passengers	Graham et al. (1997)[8]	$27,000
One-time Doppler ultrasound screening	No screening	Asymptomatic 60-year-old men with a low prevalence of >59% carotid stenosis	Derdeyn et al. (1996)[9]	$56,000
Continuing care from a community psychiatric nurse	Continuing care from a general practitioner	Patients with a range of nonpsychotic problems	Revicki et al. 1997[5]	$69,000
Dual air bags	Driver-side air bag only	Driving population and passengers	Graham et al. (1997)[8]	$69,000
MRI scan of head	CT scan of head	35-year-old women presenting with single episode of asymmetric neurological symptom suggesting possible neurological disorder	Mushlin et al. (1997)[10]	$110,000
Annual Doppler ultrasound screening	One-time Doppler ultrasound screening	Asymptomatic 60-year-old men with a low prevalence of >59% carotid stenosis	Derdeyn et al. (1996)[9]	Dominated

Source: Adapted from ref. 11.

health care coverage.[12] New treatments must now compete with each other and existing treatments and demonstrate greater cost-effectiveness before being included on formularies in these countries. Decision makers can list interventions in a league table, which ranks them according to the magnitude of their ICERs (see Table 14.1). In comparing the results of a number of independent CUAs, it is important that key methodological features are standardized to ensure a level playing field. These include the choice of discount rate, the method of estimating utility values for health states, the range of costs and consequences considered, and the choice of comparison treatments.[2,13]

Once comparable study results are ranked, decision makers have three options. They can (1) begin with a limited budget and purchase the most cost-effective interventions for a population first, working their way down the league table until the budget is exhausted; (2) determine a cost-effectiveness threshold and then provide all cost-effective interventions to a population; or (3) use the cost-effectiveness data available in a league table as one of many factors to consider in deciding on which interventions to provide. Until CUAs are fully standardized, the latter is the only feasible option open to health care decision makers. However, the second also garners a great deal of attention as researchers and decision makers attempt to determine the cost-effectiveness threshold.

Generally, interventions with an ICER less than $50,000/QALY are considered to be cost effective, but there is a great deal of disagreement about this benchmark. The most common source supporting this threshold seems to be Medicare's decision in the 1970s to cover dialysis in patients with chronic renal failure at an ICER within this range.[14] Many feel that the true cost-effectiveness threshold is actually much higher, and ICERs ranging from $50,000 to $100,000/QALY are today commonly described as also being cost effective. The statistical value-of-life literature, which uses willingness to pay surveys and revealed-preference approaches to infer the value of life from actual behavior (see Chapter 17), suggests that interventions with ICERs as high as $200,000/QALY should also be considered cost effective.[15]

In summary, a CUA measures outcomes in QALYs, a composite measure that incorporates both morbidity and mortality. The use of uniform outcome measures facilitates comparisons across programs; various health care interventions can then be compared in a league table to determine which one generates the greatest utility for a given monetary investment (see Table 14.1). However, there are a number of measurement issues that must be considered in constructing both utility weights and quality-of-life measures, and these will be explored in Chapters 15 (Utility Assessment) and 16 (Measuring Health-Related Quality of Life within Clinical Research Studies).

References

1. Drummond MF, O'Brien BJ, Stoddart GL, Torrance GW. *Methods for the Economic Evaluation of Health Care Programmes.* New York: Oxford University Press; 1997.
2. Gold MR, Siegel JE, Russell LB, Weinstein MC. *Cost-effectiveness in Health and Medicine.* New York: Oxford University Press; 1996.
3. Gage BF, Cardinalli AB, Albers GW. Cost-effectiveness of warfarin and aspirin for prophylaxis of stroke in patients with non-valvular atrial fibrillation. *JAMA.* 1995;274:1839–1845.
4. Sisk JE, Moskowitz AJ, Whang W. Cost-effectiveness of vaccination against pneumococcal bacteremia among elderly people. *JAMA.* 1997; 278:1333–1339.
5. Revicki DA, Brown RE, Keller MB. Cost-effectiveness of newer antidepressants compared with tricyclic antidepressants in managed care settings. *J Clin Psychiatry.* 1997;58:47–58.
6. Tsevat J, Duke D, Goldman L. Cost-effectiveness of captopril therapy after myocardial infarction. *J Am Coll Cardiol.* 1995;26:914–919.
7. Nord E, Wisloff F, Hjorth M. Cost-utility analysis of melphalan plus prednisone with or without interferon–α2b in newly diagnosed multiple myeloma. *PharmacoEconomics.* 1997;12:89–103.
8. Graham JD, Thompson KM, Goldie SJ. The cost-effectiveness of air bags by seating position. *JAMA.* 1997;278:1418–1425.
9. Derdeyn CP, Powers WJ. Cost-effectiveness of screening for asymptomatic carotid atherosclerotic disease. *Stroke.* 1996;27:1944–1950.
10. Mushlin AI, Mooney C, Holloway RG. The cost effectiveness of magnetic resonance imaging for patients with equivocal neurological symptoms. *Int J Technol Assess Health Care.* 1997;13:21–34.
11. Neumann, PJ. The Cost-Effectiveness Analysis Registry. Harvard Center for Risk Analysis. Available at: http://www.hsph.harvard.edu/cearegistry/data/panel_worthy.pdf. Accessed July 10, 2005.
12. George B, Harris A, Mitchell A. Cost-effectiveness analysis and the consistency of decision making: Evidence from pharmaceutical reimbursement in Australia (1991 to 1996). *PharmacoEconomics.* 2001;19:1103–1109.
13. Drummond M, Torrance G, Mason J. Cost effectiveness league tables: More harm than good? *Soc Sci Med.* 1993;37:33–40.
14. Neumann PJ. *Using Cost-effectiveness Analysis To Improve Health Care: Opportunities and Barriers.* Oxford: Oxford University Press; 2005:157–158.
15. Hirth RA, Chernew ME, Miller E, Fendrick AM, Weissert WG. Willingness to pay for a quality-adjusted life year: In search of a standard. *Medical Decision Making.* 2000;20:332–342.

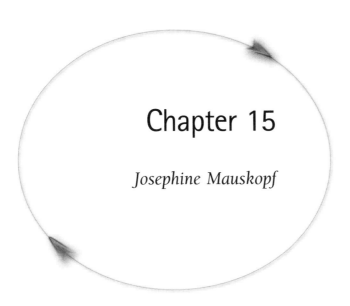

Chapter 15

Josephine Mauskopf

Utility Assessment

Most methods of measuring health-state utility are based on a definition of utility as a measure of an individual's relative preferences for different health states compared to death and perfect health. Generally utility is measured in units between 0 and 1 with 0 representing death (or the worst possible health outcome) and 1 representing perfect health. There are several different methods that can be used to measure utility and there is no consensus as to which method should be used. In this chapter, we will describe several of the most commonly used methods and summarize their strengths and weaknesses. Before we present the methods that are used to measure the utility for different health states, we will briefly describe the way that these measures are used in economic evaluations for new health care interventions.

Use of Utility Weights in Cost Effectiveness Analyses

The economic evaluation of a new health care intervention requires a comparison of the changes in costs and benefits attributable to the new intervention from the perspective either of society or of different health care decision makers. Economic evaluations are used both to compare the value of alternative treatments for a single health condition as well as to compare the value of treatments for different health conditions. The latter comparison is especially important when the total expenditures on health care are subject to a budget limit.

In order to compare the value of interventions for different health conditions, it is necessary that the measures for costs and benefits are ones that can be used for any health condition and any type of health care intervention. Costs are always measured in currency units and are the same for interventions for different conditions. However, the benefits associated with a new intervention may be different for different health conditions and different types of interventions—for one condition the main benefit from a new intervention could be to reduce mortality (e.g., surfactant prophylaxis or rescue therapy for respiratory distress syndrome for very premature infants), while for another condition the main benefit could be to reduce pain (e.g., a new migraine drug), and for another to reduce the number of cases of a disease (e.g., influenza vaccination).

To compare the value of interventions for different conditions it is critical that we have a measure that is able to map all of these very different benefits from new health care interventions into a single unit of measure. The unit that is commonly accepted as the best measure of benefit from a new health care intervention is the *quality-adjusted life year* (QALY). Quality-adjusted life years are computed by applying measures of relative levels of well being or quality in different health states (the utility weights) to the health states experienced in each remaining year of life. QALY gains from a new intervention are based on the observation that health gains from new interventions may have two elements–a change in the expected number of remaining life-years and a change in the health states of some or all of those remaining life years. Quality-adjusted life years with different interventions are computed by adjusting estimates of a typical patient's remaining life expectancy by a measure of the utility (the utility weight) associated with the health state(s) in which the person spends each remaining year of life with each intervention. Figure 15.1 gives an example of the calculation of QALY's gained for new interventions for an acute illness (influenza) and for a chronic illness (HIV infection).

Using utility weights to estimate QALYs requires three assumptions.[1] (1) Utility weights should be based on individual's preferences rather than based on psychometric methods that focus on the measurement of the level of health status rather than on the measurement of individual's relative preferences for different levels of health status. (2) Utility weights must also be measured on an interval scale in which equal intervals have the same value wherever they occur on the scale. This is because a QALY, as generally calculated, does not distinguish between a change in utility from 0.8 to 1 and a change in utility from 0.2 to 0.4. (3) Finally, the utility weights should be anchored on a scale from 0 (death) to 1 (perfect health). All the methods for estimating health-state utility weights that are described in this chapter attempt to satisfy these three assumptions.

Utility Assessment Methods

There are four methods that are commonly used to estimate the utility or preference weights associated with alternative health states: visual analogue scales (VAS), standard gamble (SG) lotteries, time trade-off (TTO) questionnaires, and utility function estimates. Each of these methods will be described in this chapter. They will be illustrated by examples and their advantages and disadvantages discussed.

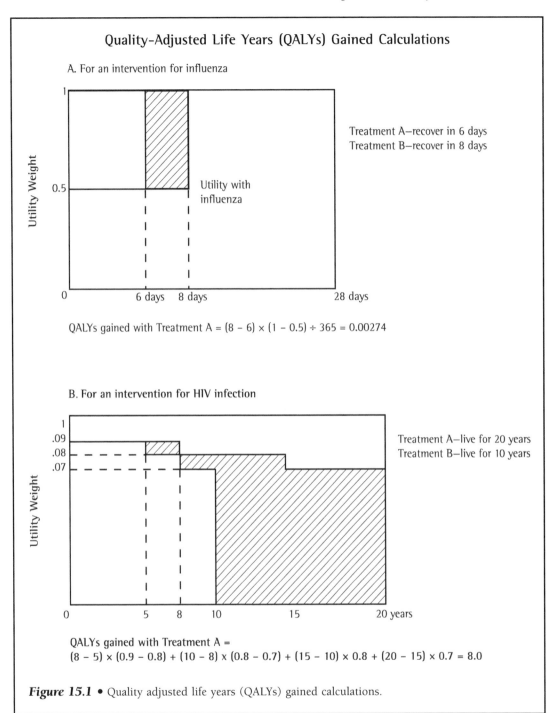

Figure 15.1 • Quality adjusted life years (QALYs) gained calculations.

Visual Analogue Scales

Visual analogue scales (VAS) for estimating utility weights are the simplest method to understand and to implement. This type of scale simply presents a line with numbers between 0 and 1 or between 0 and 100 with labels for perfect health at 1 and death or worst imaginable health state at 0 and asks the respondent to mark on the line the position between these two extremes which corresponds to their relative preferences for a specific health state. The person may be asked to mark where on the line their current health condition is located and/or to mark on the line the location for several hypothetical health states that are described to them. Figure 15.2 gives an example of scores derived using a VAS.

Visual analogue scales have been included in clinical trials for new health care interventions very frequently since they are simple to explain to clinical investigators and patients and quick to complete. They also produce values that are sensitive to changes in health states. In addition, the values for different health states ranging in severity and impact tend to use up all the space between 0 and 1.

However, strength of preference is generally defined in terms of tradeoffs—how much of one thing an individual is willing to give up in return for something else. The VAS does not explicitly ask for preference trade-offs among different health states—but rather asks for subjects to indicate the relative value of that health state compared to death and perfect health. Since there is general agreement that QALY calculations should use utility weights that represent individual's relative preferences for different health states,[1] equations have been developed for converting the values estimated using a VAS

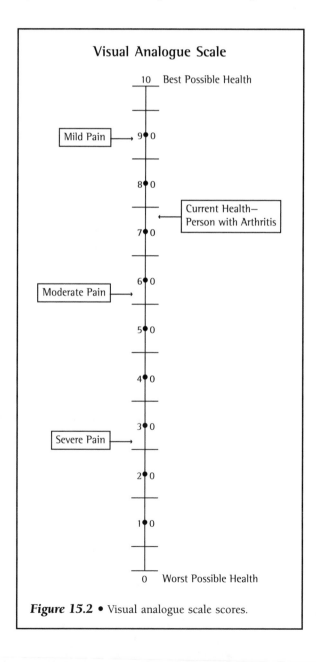

Figure 15.2 • Visual analogue scale scores.

Conversion of VAS Scores to Utility Weights

299 people with HIV infection provided both VAS scores and utility scores based on relative preferences

Using these data, two equations were estimated:

- Utility Weight = $1 - (1 - VAS)^{1.6}$
- Utility Weight = $0.44\ VAS + 0.49$

Both fit the data well

Figure 15.3 • Equation for converting visual analogue scale (vas) scores for HIV infection into utility weights based on relative preferences.[2]

---

to utility weights representing relative preferences.[2-6] Figure 15.3 gives an example of how these equations were developed by Mrus et al.[2]

Standard Gamble Lottery

There are two measures of utility that are generally considered to measure relative preferences for different health states directly and that are most commonly used to compute quality-adjusted life years. These are the standard gamble (SG) lottery and the time trade-off (TTO) questionnaire.

A typical SG lottery asks a person to choose between experiencing a specific health state with certainty for the rest of their life and a lottery, usually described as a medical intervention, with two possible outcomes, an immediate return to perfect health with probability p or immediate death with probability (1-p). The probabilities of experiencing each of these two lottery outcomes are changed until the person is indifferent between the specific health state with certainty and the lottery. The utility weight for the certain health state is assumed to equal the probability p, for perfect health, that makes the subject indifferent between the certain outcome and the probabilistic outcome based on the following expected utility calculation:

$$U(\text{Certain Health State}) = p \cdot U(\text{Perfect Health}) + (1 - p) \cdot U(\text{Death})$$
$$U(\text{Certain Health State}) = p \cdot (1) + (1 - p) \cdot (0) = p$$

Standard gamble lotteries can be interviewer administered or administered via a computer.[7,8] Generally a warm up exercise will be used first to familiarize the respondents with the exercise before the SG lottery is given.[9] The specific health state used in the SG lottery can either be the person's current health state or it can be a hypothetical health state. All the health states (i.e., the specific health state, death, and perfect health) are assumed to continue for the person's remaining expected lifetime. Figure 15.4 and Table 15.1 give examples of SG utility estimates.

The main advantage of the SG lottery method is that it gives estimates of the relative preferences for different health states using a method that is consistent with expected utility theory and thus has a sound basis in economic theory.[10,11]

There are several problems with the SG lottery method. The main problems are that it is more difficult to complete than the VAS and that people may find the risk of death to be unacceptable whatever its probability. This is particularly a problem for acute conditions where a full recovery is expected. Generally, for such conditions, respondents will not take any risk of death in the lottery.

Standard Gamble Lottery Question

A computer interview was used with screens like the one shown below. The interview started with a screen showing the lottery probability of achieving perfect health with treatment as 99% and, if the respondent chose to undergo treatment at that value, reduced the lottery probability of perfect health until the respondent chose either to "remain in the current condition" or that both options were "equally acceptable." The probability of achieving perfect health at this point was used to calculate the SG utility weight.

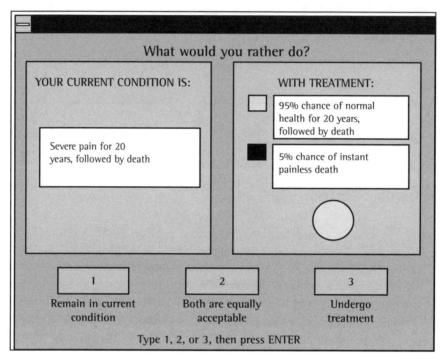

Results

Utility weight for mild pain = 0.73

Utility weight for severe pain = 0.47

Figure 15.4 • Standard gamble lottery question and resulting utility estimates for zoster pain.

Source: Reproduced with permission from Bala MV, Wood LL, Zarkin GA, et al. Valuing outcomes in health care: a comparison of willingness to pay and quality-adjusted life years. *J Clin Epidemiol.* 1998;51:667–676.

There are two alternative approaches that have been taken to use the SG lottery to develop utility weights in such cases. The first alternative is called *chaining*.[12-16] In the first stage of the chaining approach, an SG lottery questionnaire determines the probabilities at which the respondent is indifferent between being in the short duration health state of interest with certainty and a lottery between perfect health and a worst possible nonfatal health state generally for the condition of interest for the appropriate time horizon. In the second stage, an SG lottery determines the utility of the same worst possible health state used in the first lottery by assuming that it is now a certain outcome and will last for the person's remaining lifetime and determines the indifference point between it and a lottery for immediate death or perfect health. At the end of the chaining procedure, an acute health state has been translated into a utility weight on the 0 to 1 scale where 0 is the utility of death and 1 the utility of perfect health by using the standard gamble lottery method twice. Figure 15.5 gives an example of the

Table 15.1
Standard Gamble Utility Weights for Schizophrenia Including Multiple Symptom and Side Effects Descriptors

Respondents were first asked to score a series of schizophrenia symptom scenarios using a visual analogue scale and then to complete a standard gamble question asking them to give the risk of death they would accept to live without each health condition using a computer interview that included video illustration of each scenario.

The VAS and SG scores were computed for the schizophrenia symptoms scenarios both without and with common drug side effects.

Utility Weights for Schizophrenia Symptom Scenarios Without Drug Side Effects

Clinical Description of Schizophrenia Health State based on PANSS items	Mean Standard Gamble Utility Weight
Mild symptoms	0.88
Moderate with negative dominance of symptoms	0.76
Moderate with positive and negative symptoms	0.75
Severe with negative dominance of symptoms	0.65
Severe with positive and cognitive symptoms	0.66
Severe with negative and cognitive symptoms	0.56
Severe with positive dominance of symptoms	0.63
Extremely severe symptoms	0.43

Factor by Which Each Utility Weight for the Symptom Scenarios Should Be Multiplied in the Presence of a Drug Side Effect

Common Drug Side Effect	Multiplicative Disutility Factor
Orthostatic hypotension	0.912
Weight gain	0.959
Tardive dyskinesia	0.857
Pseudoparkinsonianism	0.888
Akathisia	0.898

Source: Lenert et al., 2004.

estimation of utility weights using a chaining method. It should be noted, however, that researchers who have compared the utility obtained for a chronic condition using a two-step chaining processes with direct elicitation using an SG lottery have shown inconsistent results raising some questions about the validity of the chaining method.[17]

An alternative approach for dealing with an acute health state is to assume that the acute health state will last for the person's remaining lifetime. The health state utility can then be estimated using a single standard gamble lottery questionnaire. The zoster pain utility assessment described above used this approach.[9] Both methods for estimating utility weights for acute conditions could result in estimates of the utility weights that are biased upwards if people assign higher utility weights (a lower disutility) to health states when they last for a long time and when one of the alternatives in the lottery is immediate death.

Chained Estimate of Utility

Fourteen different health states for ADHD were defined, each lasting 1 month, based on different combinations of:

- Behavior during the day
- Social well-being
- Attributes of the medicine (doses per day, school dose needed, daily behavior swings because of wearing off)
- Adverse events from the medicine (insomnia, upset stomach, headache, loss of appetite, slightly nervous or jumpy)

The respondents first ranked 14 states in order of severity using a visual analogue scale.

Then raw standard gamble (Raw SG) utility estimates were obtained from the respondents for 1 month in each state with certainty compared to a lottery with the outcomes of 1 month in perfect health or 1 month in the worst ranked state.

Next SG utility estimates were obtained from the respondent for the worst ranked state with certainty for the rest of the person's life compared to a lottery with the outcomes of a cure or immediate death.

The Adjusted SG for each of the 14 health states was computed as:

[Raw SG × (1 – SG Utility for Worst Health State)] + SG Utility for Worst Health State

Results
SG Utility for worst health state lasting a lifetime = 0.66
Current health state – Raw SG = 0.72; Adjusted SG = [0.72 × (1 – 0.66)] + 0.66 = 0.91

Figure 15.5 • Chained estimate of utility weights for attention deficit hyperactivity disorder (ADHD).[15]

Time Trade-Off Questionnaire

The time trade-off (TTO) utility assessment is similar to the standard gamble in that it asks the respondent to trade off life for gains in health status. In particular, the respondent is asked to assume that they are in a specific health state for their remaining lifetime and they are then asked how many years of their remaining lifetime would they give up to be returned to perfect health immediately. The utility weight is computed as the ratio of the shorter lifetime chosen for perfect health to their life expectancy in the specific health state of interest. A time tradeoff utility estimate can be obtained both for the person's current health status as well as for hypothetical health states. Figure 15.6 gives an example of the estimation of utility weights using time trade-off questions.

The TTO questionnaire has advantages and disadvantage compared to the VAS and SG methods. Compared to the VAS, the TTO method elicits preferences for different health states by requiring a trade-off between length and quality of life. The utilities may be easier to obtain for chronic conditions using the TTO than SG because the TTO does not require an iterative process with changing probabilities. However, like the SG lottery, the method is problematical for acute conditions where a person might not be willing to give up any life expectancy in exchange for an immediate return to perfect health. Similar to the SG lottery, either a chaining approach[12,20] or the assumption that the acute condition would last for the remaining lifetime has been used in a TTO questionnaires to obtain utility weights for acute conditions.

Time Trade-Off Estimates

EQ-5D includes five questions in these domains:

* Mobility
* Self-care
* Usual activities
* Pain/discomfort
* Anxiety/depression

For each area the answer can be:

* No problems
* Some problems
* Serious problems

Respondents first described their own health state using the EQ-5D questions.

They then ranked between 13 to 15 health states in order of severity using a visual analogue scale.

They were then told to imagine that they would live for 10 years in those health states and then die.

Finally, they were asked to indicate, for each of the health states how much of the 10 years they would give up if they could be restored to perfect health.

For example, if the health state over their remaining 10 years of life was: no problems with mobility and self care, and some problems with usual activities, pain/discomfort, and anxiety/depression.

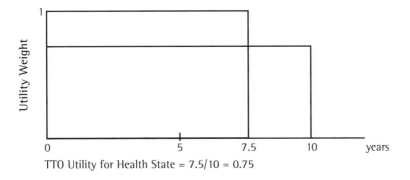

TTO Utility for Health State = 7.5/10 = 0.75

Figure 15.6 • Time trade-off (TTO) utility weights estimated for 42 general health states taken from the EQ-5D.[18,19]

Utility Function Estimates

Several researchers have developed functional relationships between overall utility weight and health states that are described by a number of health attributes. Some of these functional relationships are derived using multi-attribute utility theory[6,21,22] and others have used a more empirical approach to functional assessment.[23,24] In all cases, health is defined in multiple domains including such attributes as mobility, emotion, and pain. Within each domain, there are multiple levels of disability that are possible.

In order to develop a functional relationship between an overall utility weight and the level of disability in each domain, a subset of all the possible health states (combinations of disability levels in each domain) are selected. Each of these health states is assigned a utility weight using one of the three utility elicitation processes that we have described above, VAS, SG lottery, or TTO questionnaire. In addition, when using multiattribute utility theory (MAUT) as the basis for the functional relationship, utility weights are also estimated for each level of disability in each of the domains individually using the VAS or some other method of assigning utilities. Using regression analysis, a functional relationship is then estimated between the overall utility weight and either the utility weights for the individual domains (based on MAUT) or the disability scores for the individual domains (empirical approach). The estimated functional relationship can then be used to predict overall utility weights for all possible health states described by the domains and their disability levels.

Three examples of the estimation of utility weights using a utility function are the utility weights that have been derived for the EQ-5D,[19,23] for the SF-6D,[24] and for the Health Utility Index (HUI).[6,21,22] Figures 15.7, 15.8, and 15.9 describe how these utility weights were estimated.

Comparison of Alternative Methods for Utility Assessment

Measures of utility using the different methods to generate the estimates have been compared in several studies.[25-27] Generally, it has been found that the untransformed VAS score is more sensitive to changes in health states and gives measures that span more of the space from 0 to 1 than the SG or TTO methods. For both the TTO and the SG, the utility weights are crowded closer to 1 and thus differences

---

Utility Function Estimates for EQ-5D

Time trade-off utility estimates were derived for 42 out of the 243 possible EQ-5D health states (see Figure 15.6).

The TTO utility weights and domain levels were then used to estimate a regression equation with these parts:

- TTO Utility Weight = A + (B x Domain Level) + (C x Serious Score in Domain) + (D x Serious Problem in Any Domain)
- Using the estimated regression equation, utility weights were then estimated for the other 201 health states possible with the EQ-5D.

Figure 15.7 • Derivation of utility weights for the EQ-5D using a utility function.[19,23]

Utility Function Estimates for SF-6D

Scores from the SF36 can readily be converted into one of the 18,000 possible health states that are described using the 6 domains of the SF-6D.

A chaining approach was used to obtain standard gamble utility weights for 249 different health states.

The SG utility weights and domain levels were then used to estimate a regression equation with these parts:

- SG Utility Weight = A + (B × SF-6D Domain Level) + (C × Selected Domain Interactions)
- Using the estimated regression equation, utility weights were then estimated for all 18,000 health states possible with the SF-6D.

Figure 15.8 • Derivation of utility weights for the SF-6D using a utility function.[24]

Utility Function Estimates for HUI

Standard gamble estimation was used to generate utility weights for a small subset of the possible combination health states.

A visual analogue scale was used to assign value scores to the different levels of disability in each health domain in the HUI.

Finally, the SG utility estimates for the combination states and the domain utility weights were used to estimate a multiplicative regression equation:

$$\text{SG Utility Weight} = A \times \text{Domain 1 Utility}^{B1} \times \text{Domain 2 Utility}^{B2} \times$$
$$\text{Domain 3 Utility}^{B3} \times \ldots\ldots\text{Domain n Utility}^{Bn}$$

Using the estimated regression equation, utility weights were then estimated for the remaining combination states possible with the HUI.

Figure 15.9 • Derivation of utility weights for the HUI using a utility function.[6,22]

---

between health states are smaller than those estimated using the untransformed VAS score. The SG utilities are crowded near one probably because people are reluctant to accept mortality trade-offs. The TTO confounds time preference with health state preference by trading immediate changes in health for years of life at the end of life. The VAS values become more compressed when they are converted into utility weights using a preference equation. Figure 15.10 presents the results of studies that have compared the scores from alternative methods for utility assessment.

In addition, several studies have looked at the differences in utility weight estimates for specific health states depending on who is responding to the questionnaires.[28-31] Generally these studies have shown that those with actual experience of the condition tend to give a higher utility to the disease state than those who have not experienced the health state.[28,30,31] The recommendation for cost-effectiveness analysis by Gold et al. is that the reference case cost effectiveness analysis should use population-based utility weights.[32]

The extent to which different utility assessment methods result in similar estimates of the absolute gains or losses in utility associated with a new intervention is of greater importance for the generation of cost-effectiveness ratios than differences in the utility weights elicited using different methods or different respondents described in the previous few paragraphs. Estimates of QALYs gained or lost with new interventions depend only on the changes in utility attributable to the new intervention and not on the position on the utility scale where these changes take place. Several studies have estimated the changes in utility with changes in health status to determine whether or not the utility measures are responsive to clinical changes as well as to determine if different methods of utility assessment generate different estimates of the absolute magnitude of these changes.[33-35] These studies demonstrate that use of different measures of utility result in different estimates of the utility gains. This will in turn result in different estimates of QALYs gained and of the cost-effectiveness ratios. Figure 15.11 presents a few examples of studies that have estimated the differences in the estimated changes in utility when using alternative methods of utility assessment.

Comparison of Utility Weight Estimates Using the HUI2 and the EQ-5D in Parkinson's Disease[27]

HUI2 estimates are based on standard gamble utilities and EQ-5D estimates are based on time trade-off utilities.

Both measures are highly correlated with clinical measures of disease severity in Parkinson's disease. But mean utility values are different for 97 patients tested:

- Mean utility weight with HUI2 = 0.74
- Mean utility weight with EQ-5D = 0.58

Comparison of Utility Weight Estimates Using the VAS, TTO and the SG Methods[25]

Compared Utility Weights for Health State Defined as:

- Unable to perform some tasks at home or work
- Able to perform self care with some difficulty
- Unable to participate in leisure activity
- Often in moderate to severe pain

Mean utility weight with VAS converted using equation $1 - (1 - VAS) \ 1.6 = 0.5650$
Mean utility weight with TTO = 0.5780
Mean utility weight with SG = 0.6709

Comparison of Utility Weight Estimates Using the HUI3 or the SF-6D Methods[26]

This study compared utility scores for people at risk of sudden cardiac death.

- Mean utility weight for HUI3 = 0.61
- Mean utility weight for SF-6D = 0.58

Range of utility weight across individual patients differed between measures:

- Range of utility weights for HUI3 = −0.21 to 1.0
- Range of utility weights for SF-6D = 0.30 to 0.95

Also observed:

- For HUI3 values greater than 0.75, SF-6D values are generally lower
- For HUI3 values less than 0.4, SF-6D values are generally higher

Figure 15.10 • Difference in utility values by assessment method.[26]

Impact of Assessment Method on Gain in Utility

Pre and Post Liver Transplant:
- EQ-5D gave a 0.091 increase in utility weight
- SF-6D gave a 0.009 increase in utility weight

Treatment for Intermittent Claudication
- EQ-5D gave a 0.18 increase in utility weight
- HUI3 gave a 0.11 increase in utility weight

Pre and Post Total Hip Arthroplasty
- SG gave a 0.17 increase in utility weight
- HUI2 gave a 0.17 increase in utility weight
- HUI3 gave a 0.25 increase in utility weight

Figure 15.11 • Difference in estimates of gains in utility after treatment using different measures.[33-35]

Summary

There are several methods that have been proposed for estimating the relative preferences of individuals for different health care states including: VAS scores converted to utility weights using an equation derived from studies that have used both VAS and SG or TTO measures of utility; SG lotteries either in one or two stages depending on whether the health state is acute or chronic; TTO questionnaires either in one or two stages depending on whether the health state is acute or chronic; and utility function estimates (e.g., EQ-5D, SF-6D, and HUI1, HUI2, HUI3) derived using VAS, SG lottery, or TTO questionnaires for a subset of all possible health states.

There are several weaknesses with the current methods to estimate utility weights. First, the VAS scores are not accepted as measures of people's preferences unless they are converted to preference weights using an equation. However there is no conceptual basis for such conversions and no consensus on which equation to use. Second, SG lotteries and TTO questionnaires are not very effective for measuring utility weights for acute conditions and the different techniques used to estimate utility weights for acute conditions, using the chaining method or assuming that the acute conditions last for a lifetime, may produce measures that are biased and/or inconsistent. Finally, although utility weights are likely to vary with different health outcomes, relative preferences for different treatments are likely also to depend on mode and frequency of administration of the treatment as well as on its impact on the health outcomes. These attributes of a new treatment are rarely included in the standard measures of utility. One exception is the ADHD utility assessment described in Figure 15.5 earlier in this chapter.[15] Because of these weaknesses, the results of cost-effectiveness analyses using utility weights to estimate the QALYs gained with the new intervention should be interpreted with caution especially when comparing results across two studies that used different methods for utility assessment.

References

1. Neumann PJ, Goldie SJ, Weinstein MC. Preference-based measures in economic evaluation in health care. *Ann Rev Public Health.* 2000;21:587–611.

2. Mrus JM, Yi MS, Freedberg KA, et al. Utilities derived from visual analog scale scores in patients with HIV/AIDS. *Med Decis Making.* 2003;23:414–421.

3. Nord E. The validity of a visual analogue scale in determining social utility weights for health states. *Int J Health Plan Manage.* 1991;6:234–242.

4. Stiggelbout AM, Eijkemans MJ, Kiebert GM et al. The "utility" of the visual analogue scale in medical decision making and technology assessment. Is it an alternative to the time trade-off? *Int J Technol Assess Health Care.* 1996;12:291–298.

5. Teng TO, Lin TH. A meta-analysis of utility estimates for HIV/AIDS. *Med Decis. Making.* 2002;22:475–481.

6. Torrance GW, Furlong W, Feeny D, Boyle M. Multi-attribute preference functions: Health Utilities index. *Pharmacoeconomics.* 1995;7:503–520.

7. Lenert LA, Sturley A, Watson ME. iMPACT3: Internet based development and administration of utility elicitation protocols. *Med Decis Making.* 2002;22:464–474.

8. Lenert LA, Sturley AP, Rapaport MH et al. Public preferences for health states with schizophrenia and a mapping function to estimate utilities from positive and negative symptom scale scores. *Schizophrenia Research.* 2004;71:155–165.

9. Bala MV, Wood LL, Zarkin GA et al. Valuing outcomes in health care: a comparison of willingness to pay and quality-adjusted life years. *J Clin Epidemiol.* 1998;51:667–676.

10. Pliskin JS, Shepard DS, Weinstein MC. Utility functions of life years and health status. *Operational Res.* 1980;28:206–224.

11. Von-Neumann J, Morgenstern O. *Theory of Games and Economic Behavior.* Princeton, NJ: Princeton University Press; 1944.

12. Jansen SJ, Stiggelbout AM, Wakker PP, et al. Patients' utilities for cancer treatments: a study of the chained procedure for the standard gamble and time tradeoff. *Med Decis Making.* 1998;18:391–399.

13. Llewellyn-Thomas H, Sutherland HJ, Tibshirani R, et al. The measurement of patients' values. *Med Decis Making.* 1982;2:449–462.

14. McNamee P, Glendening S, Shenfine J, et al. Chained time trade-off and standard gamble methods: applications in oesophageal cancer. *Eur J Health Econ.* 2004;5:81–86.

15. Secnik K, Matza L, Cottrell S, et al. Health state utilities for childhood attention-deficit/hyperactivity disorder based on parent preferences in the United Kingdom. *Med Decis Making.* 2005;25:56–70.

16. Torrance GW. Measurement of health state utilities for economic appraisal. *J Health Econ.* 1986;5:1–30.

17. Oliver A. Testing the internal consistency of the lottery equivalents method using health outcomes. *Health Econ.* 2005;14:149–159.

18. Dolan P. Aggregating health state valuations. *J Health Serv Res Policy.* 1997a;2:160–165.

19. Dolan P. Modeling valuations for EuroQol health states. *Med Care.* 1997b 1095–1108.

20. Aballea S, Tsuchiya A. Seeing and doing: feasibility study towards valuing visual impairment using simulation spectacles. Discussion Paper Series. May 2004 Ref 04/4, The University of Sheffield, School of Health and Related Research (ScHARR).

21. Feeny D, Furlong W, Boyle M, Torrance GW. Multi-attribute health status classification systems. *Pharmacoeconomics.* 1995;7:490–502.

22. Feeny D, Furlong W, Torrance GW, et al. Multiattribute and single-attribute utility functions for the Health Utilities Index Mark 3 system. *Med Care.* 2002;40:113–128.

23. Greiner W, Claes C, Busschbach JJV et al. Validating the EQ-5D with time trade off for the German population. *Eur J Health Econ.* 2004. Published on-line December 22.

24. Brazier J, Roberts J, Deverill M. The estimation of a preference-based measure of health from the SF-36. *J Health Econ.* 2002;21:271–292.

25. Bleichrodt H, Johannesson M. Standard gamble, time trade-off and rating scale: experimental results on the ranking properties of QALYs. *J Health Econ.* 1997;16:155–175.

26. O'Brien BJ, Spath M, Blackhouse G, et al. A view from the bridge: agreement between the SF-6D utility algorithm and the Health Utilities Index. *Health Econ.* 2003;12:975–981.

27. Siderowf A, Ravina B, Glick H. Preference-based quality-of-life in patients with Parkinson's disease. *Neurology.* 2002;59:103–108.

28. Gabriel SE, Kneeland TS, Melton LJ, et al. Health-related quality of life in economic evaluations for osteoporosis: whose values should we use? *Med Decis Making.* 1999;19:141–148.

29. Revicki DA, Shakespeare A, Kind P. Preferences for schizophrenia-related health states: a comparison of patients, caregivers and psychiatrists. *Int Clin Psychopharmacol.* 1996;11:101–108.

30. Sung L, Young NL, Greenberg ML, et al. Health-related quality of life (HRQL) scores reported from parents and their children with chronic illness differed depending on utility elicitation method. *J Clin Epidemiol.* 2004;57:1161–1166.

31. Wild SM, Cox MH, Clark LL, et al. Assessment of health state utilities and quality of life in patients with malignant esophageal Dysphagia. *Am J Gastroenterol.* 2004;99:1044–1049.

32. Gold MR, Siegel JE, Russell LB, Weinstein MC. *Cost-Effectiveness in Health and Medicine.* New York, NY: Oxford University Press; 1996.

33. Blanchard C, Feeny D, Mahon JL, et al. Is the Health Utilities Index responsive in total hip arthroplasty patients? *J Clin Epidemiol.* 2003;56:1046–1054.

34. Bosch J, Hunink M. Comparison of the Health

Utilities Index Mark 3 (HUI3) and the EuroQol (EQ-5D) in patients treated for intermittent claudication. *Qual Life Res.* 2000;9:591–601.

35. Longworth L, Bryan S. An empirical comparison of EQ-5D and SF-6D in liver transplant patients. *Health Econ.* 2003;12:1061–1067.

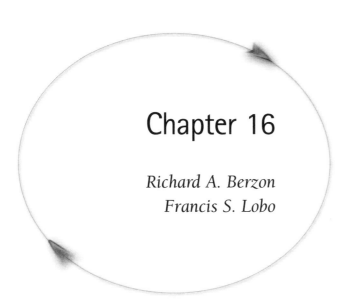

Chapter 16

Richard A. Berzon
Francis S. Lobo

Measuring Health-Related Quality of Life Within Clinical Research Studies

The field of outcomes research has widely focused on the measurement of three primary outcomes; clinical, economic, and humanistic outcomes (Figure 16.1). More recently, the U.S. Food and Drug Administration (FDA) has recommended the use of the term *patient-reported outcomes* (PROs), which serves as an umbrella term collectively describing these items. The task of assessing these outcomes has been widely undertaken in both clinical trials and observational studies. While clinical outcomes continue to remain the gold standard end-points for randomized clinical trials, information on humanistic outcomes, otherwise known as quality of life, is increasingly being collected in such studies. Especially in chronic disease states where therapeutic interventions tend to be invasive and offer limited options for a complete cure, the decision to treat may be outweighed by quality of life considerations.[1] With respect to evaluating new pharmacologic agents, this phenomenon reflects a shift away from an exclusive emphasis on safety and efficacy. It represents a new paradigm in research which, in the past, focused narrowly on laboratory and clinical indicators of morbidity and mortality. In recent years, the impact of illness and treatment on functioning and well-being are being increasingly and broadly evaluated within such study designs.[2]

This chapter discusses health-related quality of life (HRQL) and its related terms within the context of clinical trial research. HRQL questionnaires (or instruments) characterize and measure what subjects experience as a result of their receiving medical care. In this chapter, an examination of these instruments is undertaken with the understanding that there is general agreement on how HRQL is conceptualized.[3-5] As a result of this consensus on HRQL conceptualization, coupled with the usefulness and supplementation of HRQL to traditional physiologic and biologic health status assessments, these instruments are today routinely included within experimental designs.[6,7]

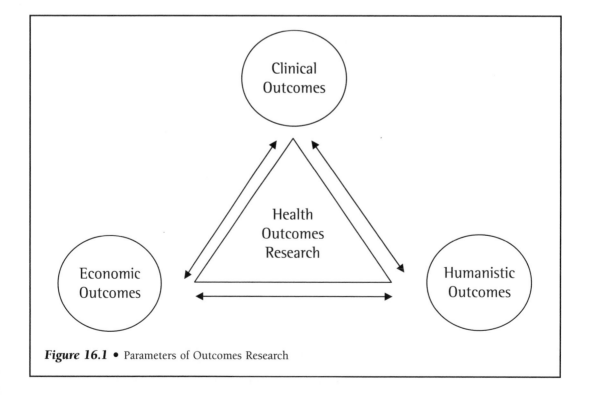

Figure 16.1 • Parameters of Outcomes Research

An underlying postulate of this chapter is that, in addition to relieving clinical symptoms and prolonging survival, a primary objective of any health care intervention is the enhancement of quality of life and well-being. Circumstances which contribute to this premise include the aging of the population and the increasing prevalence of chronic diseases; the need to evaluate health care technologies with respect to individual and societal value; and the need to recognize the patient's own perception of changes in his or her health status. Indeed, for those individuals diagnosed with a chronic condition where cure is not attainable and therapy may be prolonged, quality of life is likely to be *the* essential outcome.

Health–Related Quality of Life Construct

Quality of life (QoL) continues to be a loosely defined term, interpreted differently by researchers in different fields.[8] The World Health Organization (WHO) defines health as "not merely the absence of disease or infirmity, but a state of complete physical, mental, and social well-being."[9] This definition of health lends itself to ambiguous interpretations that need to be narrowed down, especially if such information is to be collected in clinical trials. Within the scope of a clinical trial, only those aspects of QoL which are affected by either the disease or the treatment need to be measured/assessed. Hence the term HRQL is more specific and more appropriate, as it refers to patients' appraisals of their current level of functioning compared to what they perceive to be ideal.[10] Furthermore, it encompasses the domains physical functioning, emotional and cognitive functioning, sexual functioning, general health, and social well-being, all of which are aspects of QoL that may be impacted by either the disease itself or the treatment. In recent years, there has been a slight departure from the concept of HRQL. The U.S. FDA has recommended the use of the term patient-reported outcomes (PROs) instead of HRQL (www.pro-harmonization-group.com). The term PRO refers to a host of outcomes that are provided only by the patient. Examples of these outcomes include symptom severity, perception of daily functioning, feelings of well-being, global impressions of the impact of treatment on daily life, satisfaction with treatment, and health-related quality of life. Furthermore, PRO is more representative of the patient's perspective of the impact of the treatment, especially in clinical trials.[11]

Health Profile Measures

HRQL can be assessed with health profile (descriptive) questionnaires that are either generic or specific. These questionnaires are otherwise known as HRQL instruments. The purpose of an HRQL instrument is not merely to measure the presence of severity of symptoms of disease, but also to show how the manifestations of an illness or treatment are experienced by an individual, whether that experience is descriptive or in terms of relative preferences for various health states. An HRQL instrument may seek to measure just one domain of health (i.e., just mental health). However, many HRQL instruments tend to be multidimensional in that they measure several domains of health (i.e., the MOS Short Form-36, which measures eight domains of health.[12] Generally, each domain is represented by a separate scale, and the calculation of data from each scale produces a separate numerical value (or score) that usually is unweighted. Since a disease may affect several domains of health including mental and physical, most researchers tend to use instruments measuring multidimensional traits. Single-item questions seeking to measure general health are often used in conjunction with multidimensional questionnaires, since their isolated use generally provides information of inadequate value. Examples of such single item questions seeking to measure general health include the visual analog scale (VAS), which asks respondents to rate their health on a scale of 0 (dead) to 100 (best possible health). Other examples of general health items include the frequently asked question:

How would you describe your overall health?

a. Excellent
b. Very good
c. Good, satisfactory
d. Poor

Within a clinical trial, HRQL questionnaires can be used to evaluate health care treatments to assess an agent's clinical efficacy and impact on domains of a patient's HRQL. The need for specific information by the decision maker(s), whether the decision maker is a clinician, a policymaker, or someone else, often determines the type of instrument(s) required for the experimental design. Both generic and specific health profile instruments have advantages and disadvantages and must be evaluated within the context of the needs of the particular study.

Generic Instruments

Generic instruments seek to measure HRQL regardless of illness or the condition of the population being assessed. They are often used to survey the general population which is comprised of people who normally have good health. Thus, when used in a population with a particular disease or health condition, they help anchor the HRQL of these patients against that of the general population. This information is extremely important for decision-makers, as it helps to put into perspective the health of patients with a particular disease or ailment. They also allow meaningful comparisons to be made across conditions and interventions but may not focus adequately on the area of interest for a specific intervention.

A generic health profile instrument should permit a subject to assess his or her ability to perform everyday activities across a broad range of domains. Primary HRQL domains include physical, social, and cognitive functioning, role activities, and emotional well-being.[12,13] How a subject feels about the performance of each of those activities may be assessed separately by measuring satisfaction for each domain. Alternatively, overall well-being (life satisfaction) across all domains may be assessed by means of a global question. Such as, "On a scale of 1 to 10, how would you rate your overall well-being." As is evident, the perspective of the patient is the essential component of the HRQL construct. Generic instruments need not be descriptive; alternatively, they can assess patient preferences (usually referred to as utilities).[14]

Descriptive measures are based on a psychometric approach; they are designed to provide separate scores for the key dimensions of health and a single unitary expression of health status as a global index or utility score.[15] Such utility scores are generally measured on a 0.0 to 1.0 scale, in which 0.0 is the quality of life associated with death and 1.0 is the quality of life associated with perfect health. Combining utility units with the cost of an intervention will result in a cost-utility analysis, with the utility expressed as quality adjusted life years (QALYs). Examples of generic instruments and their brief descriptions are provided below.

1. Medical Outcomes Study Short Form-36 (SF-36)

The SF-36, one of the most widely used health status questionnaires, was a product of the work by RAND and the Medical Outcomes Study (MOS) group.[12] This is a 36-item questionnaire which measures 8 domains of health including physical functioning, role-physical, bodily pain, general health perceptions, vitality, social functioning, role-emotional, and mental health. The 8 scales can also be summarized into 2 summary scores; the physical health summary (PHS) score and the mental health summary (MHS) score.

One of the major advantages of using the SF-36 is that can be self-administered and is relatively easy to complete. The reliability and validity of the SF-36 scales have also been widely established in the literature.[16,17] There have been several attempts to elicit preference scores or utilities from the SF-36, which are extremely useful for the purposes of cost-utility analyses.[18-21] The SF-36 has been translated and adapted in 29 countries. Furthermore, the SF-36 has been replicated across 24 different patient groups from various socioeconomic situations and diagnosis.[22] The SF-36 has its fair share of advantages and disadvantages. Its advantages include the fact that it is possible to compare results across studies and populations and interpret guidelines that are essential to determining the clinical, economic, and social relevance of differences in health status and outcomes. Because it is short, the SF-36 can be reproduced in a questionnaire with ample room for other more precise general and specific measures. Numerous studies have adopted this strategy and have illustrated the advantages of supplementing it.[23-25] More importantly, the SF-36 can be self-administered and has been cross-translated into at least 22 different languages. On the other hand, the disadvantages of the SF-36 are its broad applicability and generic nature, which may limit its relevance when applied to a specific patient population. Also, the percentage of floor (proportion of respondents with a score of 0) and ceiling effects (proportion of respondents with a score of 100) is another factor which might limit the use of the SF-36. Generally, it is preferred that these effects do not exceed 10%.

2. The EuroQoL (EQ-5D)

The EQ-5D is a product of the work by the EuroQoL group out of the United Kingdom.[26,27] It is comprised of five dimensions of health: mobility, self-care, usual activities, pain/discomfort, and anxiety/depression. In addition to these dimensions, respondents are also asked to rate their health on a vertical visual analog scale, which is scored from 0–100, 0 being the worst imaginable health state and 100 being the best imaginable health state. There are three possible responses to the five dimensions of health ranging from "no problems" to "some/moderate problems" to "extreme problems." The EQ-5D is generally self-administered and can be completed in a span of 2–5 minutes. Based on the responses across the five dimensions, every subject's health status is assigned a preference value from a population-based valuation system. Thus, the EQ-5D may be easily incorporated into a cost-utility analysis which requires patient preferences as a part of the denominator (generally, quality adjusted life years or quality adjusted life expectancy).

Disease or Condition-Specific Instruments

Disease or condition-specific instruments focus on dimensions of health specifically affected by a particular disease. Hence, they are likely to be more sensitive to changes in a particular disease state. They also are more sensitive to changes in health status as a function of therapeutic interventions. However, they are not comprehensive and are not conducive to across-condition comparisons; thus, limiting their use for certain populations. Specific measures continue to be generated, and guidelines for their development are readily available.[28-31] If a decision is made to construct a new disease-specific instrument, time and resources must be made available at an early state in the protocol development process (that is, as soon as phase I clinical data are available and it appears likely that such instrument development is warranted) to assure that the work is completed in a timely fashion. Condition-specific instruments very often need to be assessed for the reliability and validity of their scales. Hence, it is a common practice in clinical trials to use generic scales in conjunction with disease specific scales. Condition-specific scales have been used very often in diseases such as HIV (e.g., the MOS-HIV), arthritis (the Arthritis Impact Measurement Scale), and cancer (the EORTC QLQ-C30) among others.

1. Medical Outcomes Study–Human Immunodeficiency Virus

The MOS-HIV was developed by Wu and colleagues in response to a need for a brief HRQL instrument for multicenter clinical trials in AIDS.[31,32] The MOS-HIV is a brief, comprehensive health status measure containing 35 questions that measure 10 dimensions of health: general health perceptions, pain, physical functioning, role functioning, social functioning, energy/fatigue, mental health, health distress, cognitive function, and quality of life. A single item is also included to assess health transition. Subscales of the MOS-HIV are scored as summated rating scales on a 0 to 100 scale; again, higher scores indicate better health. In addition to these subscales, 2 summary scores can be generated: physical health summary and mental health summary scores. These are computed by transforming scores into a standardized scale with a mean of 50 and a standard deviation of 10. This enables the comparison of HIV patients in a particular clinical trial with the HIV patient populations in which the MOS-HIV was originally developed. The instrument takes approximately 5 minutes to complete and can be self-administered.

2. EORTC Core Quality of Life Questionnaire

The EORTC QLQ-C30 is designed to measure cancer patients' physical, psychological, and social functions. The questionnaire is composed of both multi-item scales and single items. The QLQ-C30 incorporates nine multi-item scales: five functional scales (physical, role, cognitive, emotional, and social) and three symptom scales (fatigue, pain, and nausea and vomiting); as well as a global health and quality of life scale. Responses to most items are captured on a four- to seven-point Likert scale, and overall dimension scores are scored from 0–100. Several single-item symptom measures are also included. The average time for completion is about 10–11 minutes.[33,34]

To further contrast health profile and preference weighted measures, one observes that descriptive questionnaires provide disaggregated measures of changes in patient functional status and satisfaction attributable to the intervention under study. *Individual* patient concerns and intervention effects are grouped into separate domains of patient function and satisfaction. On the other hand, patient preference questionnaires focus on *society* as a whole and the societal allocation of health care resources. Preference weighted measures assign a single aggregated score to changes in health status based on patient relative preferences, and allow comparison of the impact of an intervention on HRQL to other treatments for the same condition and/or to other treatments for different conditions.

Patient preference questionnaires share a disadvantage with health profile measures: they may not be responsive to small but important clinical changes experienced by the patient. In addition, patient-derived utilities can vary depending on how they are obtained—that is, measuring patient preferences via the different methodologies (standard gamble, time trade-off, or use of a rating scale) can lead to differences in scores. The resulting discrepancies in scores raise questions about the validity of any single measurement.[35,36] <AQ1>

In the final analysis, important information for health care decision making is provided by both health profile and patient preference measures. Within a clinical trial, therefore, a case can often be made to collect HRQL data in both aggregated and disaggregated forms.[37] Findings from the use of these instruments address the need for broader, more sensitive patient-based outcomes, while the integration of treatment and disease efforts that results from their use enables patients and other decision makers to consider the trade-offs that are unique to the specific illness under study.[31]

HRQL Assessment Within Clinical Trials

A clinical trial is an important medium through which treatment efficacy can be determined, and key variables within a trial's protocol inform and guide the selection of an appropriate HRQL instrument. Principal clinical trial variables include the study population, the intervention, and the clinical trial design.[38,39] The study population's demographics, its age, gender, and educational level, for example, as well as its level of illness must be considered prior to selecting an instrument. As an example, a cohort of extremely ill persons will have greater difficulty than a cohort of moderately ill persons in completing a self-administered HRQL measure. This situation may influence the integrity of the data, especially the degree to which data may be found to be missing. And so, the manner by which a questionnaire is administered should be carefully considered.[32] Options include self-administration, interviewer-administration, telephone-administration, and employing surrogate responders.[40]

The treatment regimen should be understood within the context of the other ongoing mitigating influences, such as time itself. For example, the immediate effects of coronary artery bypass graft surgery on most HRQL domains will be negative. However, 6 months after the operation, patients will undoubtedly appreciate an increase in their quality of life associated with reductions in chest pain, shortness of breath, and fatigue. Therefore, the timing of quality of life assessments is critical.

The clinical trial design should be considered with respect to issues of practicality. For example, if the trial is very complex and the patients are very ill, then the study's staff may be especially burdened. In such a case, the HRQL measure that is selected should not unduly contribute to that burden. However if HRQL is the primary endpoint, then patient and staff time should be directed to that end. As an example, when comparing two equally efficacious oncology agents, HRQL may be considered to be the critical outcome variable, and patient and staff time and energies should reflect that design. Regardless of the nature of the endpoint, the selected questionnaire should be brief and simple to complete.

The phase of the trial in which HRQL should be introduced is based on expert judgment. In small-scale phase II trials, HRQL may seem unimportant. However, should dramatic differences in clinical outcomes become evident at an early state in a treatment's evaluation, investigators may decide it is unethical to randomize patients in future trials.[40] Piloting (that is, pretesting the measure on the specific population that is to be enrolled in the trial) HRQL measures in phase II clinical trials is, therefore, a strategy that some investigators consider to gain initial insights into the intervention. Evaluation of these data from the pilot study can demonstrate both the feasibility of undertaking HRQL assessment later and the extent to which the study's design may require modification to accommodate it.

Examples of the use of HRQL instruments in the field of HIV are provided in Table 16.1. The MOS-HIV is being increasingly used in phase-2 and phase-3A/B clinical trials assessing the safety and efficacy of novel antiretroviral agents. Highly active anti-retroviral therapy (HAART) is the standard treatment practice for HIV patients, which involves the combination of multiple anti-HIV agents. Due to the combination of three or more anti-retroviral agents, therapy may involve a number of unpleasant side effects as well the burden associated with taking multiple pills. Therefore, once the decision is made to initiate therapy, the primary goals of antiretroviral therapy are to:

- Reduce HIV-related morbidity and mortality
- Improve quality of life
- Restore and preserve immunologic function
- Maximally and durably suppress viral load.

With the guidelines of therapy emphasizing an improvement in quality of life, increasing attention is being paid to this dimension of care in clinical trials. Examples of such clinical trials for anti-retroviral agents are provided in Table 16.1. In each, the MOS-HIV was the primary HRQL outcomes studied.

Evaluation Of HRQL Instruments

Psychometrics, the science of assessing the measurement characteristic of scales, is used to evaluate HRQL instruments. Psychometric properties for which an instrument should be evaluated include reliability, validity, and responsiveness (that is, sensitivity to clinically significant changes over time). Should an instrument not meet minimum recognized standards for measurement as defined by the literature (see, for example, numerous articles contained within Spilker 1996[49]), data from its use are likely to be considered questionable because of a perceived bias. Any HRQL questionnaire being considered for a particular clinical study should, if at all possible, be critically reviewed *prior* to its use in the study if results are to be taken as credible.

Reliability, validity, and responsiveness should be well understood prior to determining whether an instrument is psychometrically robust. Reliability reflects the extent to which an instrument yields reproducible and consistent results each time it is used under the same condition with the same subjects. The more reliable a measure is, the lower the element of random error. A measure found to be unreliable is not dependable. The reliability of an instrument is normally assessed in two ways: internal reliability/consistency and test-retest reliability.

Internal reliability reflects the homogeneity of items measuring a specific health domain and is normally measured using Cronbach's alpha coefficient. An alpha value of 0.70 or above is necessary to call a scale internally consistent; however, in general it is optimal to have alpha coefficients above 0.85.[50] Cronbach's alpha coefficients closer to a value of 1.0 are indicative of higher levels of homogeneity between the items. This also means that a greater level of confidence can be attributed the items constituting the domain under investigation. However, in instances where alpha coefficients of >0.95 are reported, caution should be exercised as it could possibly indicate that several of the items are in fact measuring the same thing.

Test-retest reliability is a measure of an instrument's ability to produce data that are consistent or stable over time. It is normally determined using Cohen's Kappa or Pearson's or Spearman's correlation coefficient. Normally, levels in excess of 0.6 indicate adequate test-retest reliability.[51,52] This test-retest reliability is assessed by applying the measure to the same population at different points in time under the same conditions and looking at the statistical association between the two sets of results.

Validity is defined as the extent to which an instrument measures what it is supposed to measure and does not measure what it is not supposed to measure. The concept refers to nonrandom or systematic measurement error. Of the several different types of validity, *construct validity* is especially

Table 16.1
Application of the MOS-HIV in Clinical Trials

Author	Scott-Lenox (1998)[42]
Purpose	Assessment of the impact of treatment with zidovudine plus lamivudine or zalcitabine on HRQL in patients with HIV
Number of Patients	254 HIV-positive patients (CD4+ 100–300 cells/mm^3)
HRQL Measures Used	MOS-HIV administered at baseline and weeks 16, 32, and 52
Results	Statistically significant differences across treatment groups in mean change scores on the physical functioning, role functioning, and vitality scales, with stable or increased (improved) scores in the zidovudine plus lamivudine 150 mg group and decreased scores in the zidovudine plus zalcitabine and zidovudine plus lamivudine 300 mg groups for most scales after a follow-up period of 36 weeks
Author	Cohen (1998)[43]
Purpose	Evaluation of the effect of ritonavir combined with reverse transcriptase inhibitor therapy on patient functioning and well-being
Number of Patients	1090 patients randomized to ritonavir and continued treatment with as many as two nucleoside agents (n = 543) or placebo and continued treatment with as many as two nucleoside agents (n = 547).
HRQL Measures Used	MOS-HIV and HIV-related symptoms scale administered at baseline and after 3 and 6 months of treatment using the <AQ>
Results	• After 3 months, statistically significant differences ($P < 0.03$) favoring the ritonavir-treated patients were seen on the physical health summary, mental health summary, and general health perceptions, social function, mental health, and energy/fatigue subscales.
	• After 6 months of ritonavir therapy, significant differences were observed on physical health and mental health summary scores ($P < 0.001$), and on measures of general health perceptions, physical function, role function, social function, cognitive function, mental health, health distress, energy/fatigue, and overall ratings of quality of life ($P < 0.01$).
Author	Revicki (1999)[44]
Purpose	Evaluation of the effect of zalcitabine or saquinavir monotherapy and combination saquinavir plus zalcitabine therapy on HRQL of HIV-infected adults
Number of Patients	940 HIV-infected patients (CD4 counts 50–300 cells/mm^3) who had discontinued zidovudine therapy randomized to one of three regimens: zalcitabine, saquinavir, or combination zalcitabine
HRQL Measures Used	MOS-HIV and VAS analyzed at baseline and weeks 24 and 48
Results	• After 24 weeks, the zalcitabine-treated patients demonstrated significantly greater decreases in PHS scores (–4.4 ± 0.6; saquinavir: –1.3 ± 0.6; zalcitabine plus saquinavir: –1.7 ± 0.6; $P < 0.0001$) and MHS scores (–2.2 ± 0.5; saquinavir: –1.0 ± 0.5; zalcitabine plus saquinavir: – 0.5 ± 0.5; $P = 0.032$) compared to saquinavir and zalcitabine plus saquinavir–treated patients.
	• Nine of 10 MOS-HIV subscales demonstrated results consistent with the primary endpoints.
	• After 48 weeks, a statistically significant difference between the saquinavir-treated groups and the zalcitabine monotherapy group was observed for PHS scores (zalcitabine: –5.8 ± 0.6; saquinavir: –4.1 ± 0.6; zalcitabine plus saquinavir: -3.5 ± 0.6; $P = 0.014$).

(continued)

Table 16.1 (cont'd)
Application of the MOS–HIV in Clinical Trials

Author	Chatterton (1999)[45]
Purpose	To assess the quality of life and treatment satisfaction after the addition of lamivudine or lamivudine plus loviride to zidovudine-containing regimens in treatment-experienced patients with HIV infection
Number of Patients	
HRQL Measures Used	MOS–HIV was self-administered during three scheduled clinic visits (baseline, week 28, and the end-of-treatment/withdrawal visit).
Results	• Statistically significant differences across treatment groups were demonstrated for the Physical and Mental Health Summary scores, and for 5 of 10 MOS–HIV subscales (physical functioning, vitality, cognitive functioning, general health perceptions, social functioning). • These differences favored the lamivudine and lamivudine plus loviride groups over the placebo group (p < 0.05). • No significant difference was found between the 3 treatment groups with regard to the percentages of patients who were satisfied with their study medication.
Author	Revicki (1999)[46]
Purpose	To evaluate treatment with zalcitabine-zidovudine, saquinavir-zidovudine, or saquinavir-zalcitabine-zidovudine on the health-related quality of life of HIV-infected adults with CD4 cell counts between 50 and 350 cells/mm^3
Number of Patients	993 HIV-infected male or female quality of life substudy patients aged 18 years or older, with CD4 cell counts between 50 and 350 cells/mm^3 naive to antiretroviral therapy or with <16 weeks of zidovudine therapy, were randomly assigned to one of three daily regimens: zalcitabine and zidovudine (ddC/ZDV), saquinavir and zidovudine (SQV/ZDV) or saquinavir, zalcitabine and zidovudine (SQV/ddC/ZDV)
HRQL Measures Used	MOS–HIV and a global visual analogue scale (VAS) score administered at baseline and 24 and 48 weeks
Results	• After 24 weeks of treatment, no statistically significant differences were observed between the three treatment groups on physical health and mental health summary scores (global test P = 0.118). • After 48 weeks of treatment, statistically significant differences among the groups were observed for physical health and mental health summary scores (global test P = 0.020); no change in physical health summary scores from the baseline were seen in the triple combination therapy, whereas the ddC/ZDV combination therapy group showed decreases from baseline in physical health summary scores (P = 0.008). • Six of the 10 individual MOS–HIV subscale scores and the VAS scores showed results consistent with the physical health summary endpoints after 48 weeks of therapy. • No statistically significant differences in baseline to 48 week changes in MOS–HIV subscale or summary scores were seen between the ddC/ZDV and SQV/ZDV groups (P > 0.05).

(continued)

Table 16.1 (cont'd)
Application of the MOS-HIV in Clinical Trials

Author	Casado, (2004)[46]
Purpose	To evaluate the study was to assess differences in health-related quality of life (HRQL) in HIV-infected naive patients treated with two HAART regimens
Number of Patients	127 patients, 63 patients were included in the ZDV/3TC/NFV arm and 64 in the ZDV/3TC/NVP arm
HRQL Measures Used	MOS-HIV questionnaire at the end of 12 months
Results	No statistically significant differences were observed at baseline in demographic and clinical variables and HRQL scores between treatment groups, except that the proportion of homosexual men was higher in the ZDV/3TC/NVP arm. There were no statistically significant differences in HRQL scores between arms at 12 months and over time; only ZDV/3TC/NVP patients showed statistically significant improvement in Physical Health Summary score ($p < 0.01$) and a trend toward a better profile in Mental Health Summary score ($p = 0.07$). Overall, patients who were treated with ZDV/3TC/NVP showed greater changes in physical dimensions and patients who were treated with ZDV/3TC/NFV showed greater changes in mental health

Author	Mukherjee (2003)[48]
Purpose	To evaluate effect of atazanavir therapy on patient QOL and utility compared to Lopinavir/ritonavir
Number of Patients	A total of 300 subjects were randomized and 290 were treated.
HRQL Measures Used	MOS-HIV and the EQ-5D were administered at baseline, week 24 and end of study
Results	Baseline scores were comparable in both treatment arms. After 24 weeks, using the criteria of two points or more to determine clinically meaningful changes in MOS summary scores, Atazanavir therapy was associated with clinically relevant improvement in mental health sub-scale (2.3 increase) vs. none in lopinavir/ritonovair arm. Using the criteria of two points or more to determine clinically meaningful changes in MOS domain scores, at week 24, atazanavir therapy was associated with clinically relevant improvement in six domains (general health, pain, mental health, energy/fatigue, health distress, and quality of life) and worsening in physical function. Lopinavir/ritonavir improved three domains (general health, health distress and quality of life). If a five-point criteria was used for domain scores, atazanavir therapy improved patients' general health, and health distress, while Lopinavir/ritonavir improved general health and quality of life.

Author	Cohen (2004)
Purpose	To assess the impact of enfuvirtide on HRQL
Number of Patients	A total of 995 treatment-experienced HIV-1–infected individuals received either self-administered enfuvirtide (90 mg twice daily) + optimized background (OB) or OB alone and had at least one follow-up visit
HRQL Measures Used	MOS-HIV questionnaire administered at baseline and at 4, 8, 16, and 24 weeks
Results	There were no significant between-group differences in any HRQL measure at baseline. Most MOS-HIV scores showed improvement in the enfuvirtide arm compared with OB alone, although only some of these were significant. Improvements in the general health scale were significantly higher in the enfuvirtide arm compared with OB alone at all post-baseline time points. No

(continued)

Table 16.1 (cont'd)
Application of the MOS–HIV in Clinical Trials

> scale or summary score for the OB arm showed a significantly greater improvement in score from baseline compared with the enfuvirtide arm, at any time point. The mental health summary score at 24 weeks was significantly higher in the enfuvirtide arm compared with OB alone. Enfuvirtide in addition to an OB regimen does not adversely affect and may improve HRQL when self-administered for up to 24 weeks by treatment-experienced, HIV-1–infected individuals.

relevant. Because in most cases no absolute criterion (that is, no gold standard) exists against which to validate an instrument, one becomes involved in collecting empirical evidence to support the inference that a particular measure has meaning. A measure of physical health may be tested against a measure of activities of daily living, with the prediction that the correlation should be positive. If this proves to be the case, it would be evidence of *convergent validity*. To the extent it can be demonstrated that the measure does not correlate with variables to which it should not be related, *discriminant validity* is made evident. For example, a measure of physical function should not be highly correlated with a measure of mental health. Another form of validity, *content validity*, refers to the adequacy with which a domain has been defined and sampled. While content validity is a more precise expression than *face validity* (which is defined by its reasonableness in representing a particular HRQL domain), the two terms are often used interchangeably.

Responsiveness is the extent to which an instrument can detect true differences within the construct being measured. It is geared towards measuring changes within patients in terms of their health status over time. To evaluate treatment efficacy, it is essential that an HRQL instrument to have demonstrated an ability to detect small but meaningful changes over time. If such information is unavailable, then the study can be designed so that at its conclusion HRQL changes can be compared with changes in clinical status, intervening health events, interventions of known or expected efficacy, or direct reports of change by patients or providers, among other items. Responsiveness in many ways confirms the validity of an instrument by checking to see if the estimated responses occurred in conjunction with changes in the patient's health status.[53] In the past, responsiveness has not received sufficient attention in the development of HRQL questionnaires; however, investigators are increasingly providing this information as part of an instrument's psychometric properties. In addition, the meaning of responsiveness statistics has become a focus of much needed research.[54-56]

Cross–Cultural HRQL Assessment

Clinical research today is international in scope, and the demand for the HRQL instruments that can be utilized in the same trial cross-nationally has dramatically increased. To date, a vast proportion of the HRQL instruments have been developed in English-speaking countries such as the U.S. and the UK. Even though reliability and validity of these instruments have been established, these psychometric properties might not translate to other countries/cultures. Beliefs and values about health differ significantly among cultures. Hence, prior to using an HRQL questionnaire in a culture that is extrinsic from the country in which it was originally developed, consideration must be given to whether the measure conforms to the target culture or nationality. Variations in such factors as perceptions of health and sickness, the interpretation of symptoms, the meaning of quality of life, and expectations for care must be understood to properly assess HRQL. Whether results from one culture can be applied to another will determine, for example, whether international HRQL data can be pooled at the conclusion of the study.[57,58]

Culturally adapting a HRQL questionnaire indicates that the language and meaning within the instrument are consistent with that of the target country.[59] The approach that has been used most commonly to translate a measure from one culture to another involves a forward/backward translation process of an original source language document into the target language. In addition, focus groups are often used for critical evaluation of the translation.[3]

Specific methodologies to ensure cross-cultural comparability of HRQL instruments include a sequential approach (examples include the Nottingham Health Profile, the SF-36 and the Sickness Impact Profile), a parallel approach (examples include the EORTC QLQ-C30 and the recently published Herpes-Specific HRQL Measure), and a simultaneous approach (examples include the WHOQOL and the recently published Migraine-Specific HRQL Measure). Guidelines for the adaptation of a measure from one cultural context to another may be found in the literature.[60,61] In short, the adapted questionnaire should be tested for cultural equivalence in patients within the target country prior to its use.[59, 62]

Collecting HRQL Data And Assuring Its Integrity

The inclusion of HRQL in clinical research yields three important results. First, it allows the investigator to characterize the impact of a given condition or disease in terms of clinically relevant humanistic attributes which are likely to be understood by the subject. Second, because HRQL domains may be independent predictors of important clinical outcomes such as treatment adherence, morbidity and condition severity, and mortality, these data may provide valuable insights into the natural history and progression of the condition or disease. And third, HRQL measurements provide data on how a treatment influences an individual's daily functioning.

Subjective evaluation underlies HRQL assessment, and its measurement is delineated by an individual's perception of how he or she functions in specified domains as influenced by his or her health status, health care, and health promoting activities. Additional aspects of HRQL that stem from this understanding and should be incorporated into its assessment are the individual's perceived health and overall well-being. While the definition excludes from measurement contextual factors that influence HRQL (for example, pain and other symptoms), these variables may play an important role in studies designed to better understand the impact of health care interventions on people's lives. Therefore, a broad range of variables should be considered in the context of their relevance to specific studies and populations. Pain, for example, while not a specific HRQL domain per se, will influence perceptions of functional status and overall life quality; therefore it may be appropriate to measure it within specific study designs.[13]

As with all data collected within a prospective clinical study, HRQL data should be captured so as to assure its quality and integrity. Missing data will often introduce bias in the analysis stage of HRQL information. Missing data occur primarily due to two reasons: patient drop-out from a trial and/or incomplete responses to self-administered questionnaires. There are two facets to missing data; either they are random or non-random in nature. If they are random, then to a large extent they can be regarded as being similar to the available data. However, if they are nonrandom in nature (in the event that there is a systematic pattern to missing data), then available patient data is not representative and will give rise to biased estimates. Fayers and Machin define two types of missing data; unit nonresponse and item nonresponse.[1] Unit nonresponses occur when a patients fails to complete an entire HRQL questionnaire. This may occur due to patient drop-out, missing HRQL forms, or late enrollments into a clinical trial. Item nonresponses occur in instances when one or more items are not completed within a HRQL questionnaire.[1]

In particular, measures of HRQL that are selected for a study should: (1) be consistent with the concept of HRQL; (2) collect data that can be reliably and validly assessed; (3) collect data that are likely to exhibit sensitivity to changes over time; and (4) collect data that account for most of the variance in a subject's rating of his or her overall well-being. Inadequate patient accrual and follow-up in trials that include HRQL instruments introduce serious bias into the analysis of these data; such bias is likely to compromise the integrity of the study and may lead to uninterpretable results. If the collection of HRQL data is deemed necessary to the conduct of a clinical study, these data should be obtained from all patients.

Patient compliance with HRQL questionnaires will be more likely if short, simple instruments are employed, if a relatively nondemanding data collection schedule is built into the protocol, and if specific individuals within the investigator's office or clinic are identified to coordinate and monitor HRQL data collection. This strategy will assure that the amount of missing data is kept to a minimum. In addition, the collection of these data should be planned around protocol-driven visits. For some study designs, the use of modes of questionnaire execution other than self-administration—such as interviewing subjects via telephone at home at a pre-arranged time—may be appropriate.

The individual designated to coordinate HRQL data collection at the study site should be thoroughly familiar with the instrument prior to its administration. The coordinator may encounter, for example, a respondent with low literacy skills or poor eyesight that makes it difficult for him or her to complete the questionnaire without assistance. In this case, HRQL questions and their answer choices can be read to the respondent, and the coordinator's familiarity with the specific questions will assure deft accomplishment of the task. However, questions that appear in the instrument should not be interpreted or reworded because the meaning of a question can be unintentionally altered in this way, introducing a bias. If, on review by a responsible individual, an item is found to be missing when the subject has completed the questionnaire, the subject should be asked if the item was intentionally unanswered. If so, refusal should be noted on the questionnaire so that these data can be analyzed separately.

The interpretation of HRQL study results hinges on translating changes in these scores into clinically meaningful terms. This translation may be undertaken using different approaches. One technique for both health profile and patient preference instruments is to compare the changes associated with the use of a new therapy with those changes associated with the use of therapies previously considered beneficial (using the same instrument). Recently, in a disease-specific health profile instrument, an attempt was made to identify the minimal important difference in a domain score which patients perceived as beneficial and which would likely mandate, in the absence of bothersome side effects and excessive cost, a change in the patient's management.[56,63]

Methods to analyze and interpret HRQL data may be found in the literature.[64-66] Three related issues, however, are particularly noteworthy. The first is that missing data of both a random and nonrandom nature will likely result from the use of HRQL instruments. The analysis of randomly missing data is generally well defined; however, methods to analyze nonrandom missing data remain in development. Fayers and Machin provide a detailed description of how to deal with missing data.[1] A description of two commonly used methods is provided below:

1. *Complete case analysis.* In this methodology, only those cases with complete data are included for the purposes of analyses. A major pitfall to such an analysis is that it biases results in favor of much

healthier patients who tend to stick through the entire clinical trial. The rule of thumb for conducting such an analysis is that the extent of missing data should be less than 5% of the patients.

2. *Imputation of missing data*. In this methodology, the missing data is replaced by imputed data from the existing data file. Methodologies for imputation include; simple mean imputation, where in the missing scale score is estimated from the means of those items that are available, and regression imputation, where the missing values are replaced by predicted values obtained by regressing the missing item on the remaining items of the scale.

The second issue related to the analysis of HRQL data is the interpretation on communication of results, given its multivariate nature. That is, not only is HRQL a multidimensional concept measured by multiple scales, but most studies are longitudinal. Separate analyses of each domain at multiple time points may make it difficult to communicate results in a meaningful fashion to clinicians and patients, while summary measures may reduce the multidimensionality of the problem without facilitating the complexity of interpretation. Weighting the items is likely to add to the intricacy of interpretation.

The third quandary related to the analysis of these data is how to integrate HRQL and survival data such that the resulting information is clinically meaningful and easily interpretable.[67]

An important aspect of HRQL that continues to be actively debated is that of the issue of statistical significance versus clinically meaningful significance. One must bear in mind that statistically significant differences do not necessarily translate into clinically meaningful differences. Statistical significance indicates that the probability of the differences is indeed true in nature rather than being attributed to chance. It does not in any way reflect the magnitude of these differences. Large sample sizes tend to exaggerate the levels of statistical significance (by lowering the p-value), which is meaningless if the differences are extremely small. The use of minimal clinically important differences (MCID) is gaining popularity due to the need to understand and inform the dynamics of the therapeutic encounter between patients and their physicians. The MCID is the smallest difference in scores for a HRQL domain from baseline to follow-up that patients perceive to be beneficial. This difference would result in a change in patient management, in the absence of side-effects and excessive costs and inconveniences.[56] The MCID provides a better interpretation of improvements/changes in quality of life since it incorporates the perspectives of both patients and their physicians.

Two approaches have been proposed for defining clinically meaningful changes, the anchor-based approach and the distribution-based approach. The anchor-based approach is often used in studies that are cross-sectional or longitudinal in nature. Anchor-based approaches compare HRQL measures to other measures or phenomena that have clinical relevance. Distribution-based approaches are based on statistical characteristics such as statistical significance, sample variation, or measurement precision. Crosby *et al.*[68] provide a detailed description of methodologies on clinically meaningful change.

Conclusion

Conceptual, methodological, and practical consideration should precede HRQL measurement within clinical research studies. Among the many considerations, those that seem especially pertinent include designing the study so that HRQL data can be collected easily without interfering with the collection of other, equally important information; selecting an appropriate instrument (health profile, patient preference, or both) for the relevant audience (clinician, patient, managed care administrator, policymaker, or other); considering the unique aspects of the study population, particularly the burden of the illness under investigation; evaluating the instrument's psychometric strengths and weaknesses; assuring data integrity and minimizing missing data through specific quality control procedures; and appraising how the HRQL data will be analyzed and interpreted prior to initiating patient accrual.

A variety of challenging issues are currently being studied. A few of those cited within this chapter include the integration of health profile measurement and patient preference weighting; the expeditious cross cultural adaptation of HRQL instruments for international trials; the analysis and meaningful interpretation of HRQL data; and the development of guidelines to evaluate the psychometric properties of HRQL questionnaires. The latter point is especially timely (if the audience for the data is a regulatory authority) because of the degree to which a measure must be identified as reliable, valid, and responsive; therefore, unbiased and credible prior to its use within a pivotal drug efficacy trial. Currently, the U.S. FDA has recommended that survival and quality of life data be accepted as key efficacy parameters for the approval of new anticancer agents; however, it is unclear which instruments will satisfy this requirement and whether the same instruments must be used across study designs.

Methods and tools to measure health-related quality of life are readily available. Those who undertake such measurement within clinical research studies must continue to publish their findings in peer review journals and debate their work in public so that those unacquainted with the discipline can become familiar with it. The scientific rigor of HRQL research, regardless of whether it is conducted within academia or within industry, will determine the extent to which the data are accepted by audiences to whom these outcomes are directed.

References

1. Fayers P, Machin D. *Quality of Life: Assessment, Analysis and Interpretation.* West Sussex, England: John Wiley and Sons Ltd.; 2000.
2. Berzon RA, Mauskopf JA, Simeon GP. Choosing a health profile (descriptive) and/or a patient-preference (utility) measure for a clinical trial. In: B. Spilker, ed. *Quality of Life and Pharmacoeconomics in Clinical Trials.* 2nd ed. Philadelphia: Lippincott-Raven; 1995.
3. Bullinger M, Power MJ, Aaronson NK, et al. Creating and evaluating cross-cultural instruments. In: Spilker B, ed. *Quality of Life and Pharmacoeconomics in Clinical Trials.* 2nd ed. Philadelphia: Lippincott-Raven; 1995:659–668.
4. Schipper H, Olweny CLM, Clinch, JJ. A mini-handbook for conducting small-scale clinical trials in developing countries. In: Spilker B, ed. *Quality of Life and Pharmacoeconomics in Clinical Trials.* 2nd ed. Philadelphia: Lippincott-Raven; 1995:669–680.
5. Moinpour CM. Measuring quality of life: an emerging science. *Semin Oncol.* 1994;21:48S–63S.
6. Cleary P. Future directions of quality of life research. In: Spilker B, ed. *Quality of Life and Pharmacoeconomics in Clinical Trials.* 2nd ed. Philadelphia: Lippincott-Raven; 1995:73–78.
7. Wilson IB, Cleary PD. Linking clinical variable with health-related quality of life. *J Am Med Assoc.* (1995);273:59–65.
8. Chumney ECG, Delinokov S, Fuldeore M, et al. What exactly do you mean by that? A summary of discrepancies in the definitions of key pharmacoeconomic and outcomes research terms: a white paper. *ISPOR Connections.* (2004);9(1):6.
9. World Health Organization. *The First Ten Years of the World Health Organization.* Geneva: WHO; 1958.
10. Cella DF, Tulsky DS. Measuring quality of life today: methodological aspects. *Oncology.* 1990;5:29–38.
11. Wiklund I. Assessment of patient-reported outcomes in clinical trials: the example of health-related quality of life. *Fund Clin Pharmacol.* 2004;18:351–363.
12. Ware JD, Sherbourne CD. The MOS 36-item short form health survey (SF-36): I. Conceptual framework and item selection. *Med Care.* 1992;30:473–483.
13. Shumaker SA, Naughton MJ. The international assessment of health-related quality of life. In: Shumaker SA, Berzon RA, eds. *The International Assessment Of Health-Related Quality Of Life: Theory, Translation, Measurement And Analysis.* Oxford: Rapid Communications; 1995:3–10.
14. Torrance GW. Utility approach to measuring health-related quality of life. *J Chronic Dis.* 1987;40:593–600.
15. Kaplan RM, Bush JW. Health-related quality of life measurement for evaluation, research and policy analysis. *Health Psychol.* 1982;1:61–80.
16. Haley SM, McHorney CA, Ware JE Jr. Evaluation of the MOS SF-36 physical functioning scale (PF-10): II. Unidimensionality and reproducibil-

ity of the Rasch item scale. *J Clin Epidemiol.* 1994;50(4):451–461.

17. McHorney CA, Ware JE Jr, Raczek AE. The MOS 36-item short-form health survey (SF-36): II. Psychometric and clinical tests of validity in measuring physical and mental health constructs. *Med Care.* 1993;31(3):247–263.

18. Fryback DG, Lawrence WF, Martin PA, Klein R, Klein BE. Predicting quality of well-being scores from the SF-36: results from the Beaver Dam health outcomes study. *Med Decision Making.* 1997;17(1):1–9.

19. Nichol MB, Sengupta N, Globe DR. Evaluating quality-adjusted life years: estimation of the health utility index (HUI2) from the SF-36. *Med Decision Making.* 2001;21(2):105–112.

20. Brazier J. Roberts J. Deverill M. The estimation of a preference-based measure of health from the SF-36. *J Health Econ.* 2002;21(2):271–292.

21. Lobo FS, Gross CR, Matthees BJ. Estimation and comparison of derived preference scores from the SF-36 in lung transplant patients. *Qual Life Res.* 2004;13(2):377–388.

22. Ware JE. The MOS 36-item short form health survey (SF-36). In: Sederer LI, Dickey, B, eds. *Outcomes Assessment in Clinical Practice.* Baltimore, MD: Williams & Wilkins; 1996.

23. Wagner AK. Gandek B. Aaronson NK. et al. (1998) Cross-cultural comparisons of the content of SF-36 translations across 10 countries: results from the IQOLA Project. International Quality of Life Assessment. Journal of Clinical Epidemiology. 51(11):925-32.

24. Kantz ME, Harris WJ, Levitsky K, Ware JE, Davies AR. Methods for assessing condition-specific and generic functional status outcomes after total knee replacement. *Med Care.* 1992;30(Suppl 5):MS240–MS252.

25. Nerenz DR, Repasky DP, Whitehouse FW, Kahkonen DM. Ongoing assessment of health status in patients with diabetes mellitus. *Med Care* 1992;30(Suppl 5):MS112–MS124.

26. The EuroQoL Group. EuroQoL: a new facility for the measurement of health-related quality of life. *Health Policy.* 1990;16(3):199–208.

27. Kind P, Dolan P, Gudex C, Williams A. Variations in population health status: results from a United Kingdom national questionnaire survey. *Br Med J.* 1998;316(7133):736–741.

28. Juniper EF, Guyatt GH, Jaeschke R. How to develop and validate a new health-related quality of life instrument. In: Spilker B, ed. *Quality of Life and Pharmacoeconomics in Clinical Trials.* 2nd ed. Philadelphia: Lippincott-Raven; 1995:49–56.

29. Leplege A, Verdier A. The adaptation of health status measures: methodological aspects of the translation procedures. In: Shumaker SA, Berzon RA, eds. *The International Assessment of Health-*

Related Quality Of Life: Theory, Translation, Measurement and Analysis. Oxford: Rapid Communications; 1995:93–101.

30. Streiner DL, Norman GR. (1989). *Health Measure Scales: A Practical Guide to Their Use.* New York: Oxford University Press; 1989.

31. Wu AW, Rubin HR. (1994). Approaches to health status measurements in HIV disease: overview of the conference. *Psychol Health.* 1994;9:1–18.

32. Wu AW, Jacobson D, Berzon RA, et al. (1997). Effect of mode of administration on medical outcomes, study health ratings, and EuroQol scores in AIDS. *Qual Life Res.* 1997;6:3–10.

33. Aaronson NK, Ahmedzai S, Bergman B, Bullinger M, Cull A, Duez NJ, Filiberti A, Flechtner H, Fleishman SB, de Haes JC, et al. The European Organization for Research and Treatment of Cancer QLQ-C30: a quality-of-life instrument for use in international clinical trials in oncology. *J Natl Cancer Inst.* 1993;85:365–376

34. Sprangers MAG, Cull A, Bjordal K, et al. The European Organization for Research and Treatment of Cancer approach to quality of life assessment: guidelines for developing questionnaire modules. *Qual Life Res.* 1993;2:287–295.

35. Guyatt G, Feeny D, Patrick D. Issues in quality of life measurement in clinical trials. *Control Clin Trials.* 1991;12:81S–90S.

36. Revicki DA, Kaplan RM. Relationship between psychometric and utility-based approaches to the measurement of health-related quality of life. In: Shumaker SA, Berzon RA, eds. *The International Assessment of Health-Related Quality Of Life: Theory, Translation, Measurement and Analysis.* Oxford: Rapid Communications; 1995:125–135.

37. Drummond, M. Quality of life measurement within economic evaluations. Paper presented at the ESRC/SHHD workshop on Quality of Life, Edinburgh, Scotland, April 27–28, 1993.

38. Gotay CC, Korn EL, McCabe MS, et al. Building quality of life assessment into cancer treatment studies. *Oncology.* 1992;6:25–37.

39. Schron EB, Shumaker SA. The integration of health-related quality of life in clinical research: experiences from cardiovascular clinical trials. *Prog Cardiovasc Nurs.* 1992;7:21–28.

40. Guyatt GH, Jaeschke R, Feeny DH, Patrick DL. Measurements in clinical trials: choosing the right approach. In: Spilker B, ed. *Quality of Life and Pharmacoeconomics in Clinical Trials.* 2nd ed. Philadelphia: Lippincott-Raven; 1995:41–48.

41. Pocock SJ. A perspective on the role of quality of life assessment in clinical trials. *Control Clin Trials.* 1991;191;12:265S–275S.

42. Scott-Lennox JA, Mills RJ, Burt MS. Impact of zidovudine plus lamivudine or zalcitabine on health-related quality of life. *Annals*

*Pharmacother.*1998;32(5):525–530.

43. Cohen C, Revicki DA, Nabulsi A, Sarocco PW, Jiang P. A randomized trial of the effect of ritonavir in maintaining quality of life in advanced HIV disease. Advanced HIV Disease Ritonavir Study Group. *AIDS.* 1998;12(12):1495–1502.

44. Revicki DA, Moyle G, Stellbrink HJ, Barker C. Quality of life outcomes of combination zalcitabine-zidovudine, saquinavir-zidovudine, and saquinavir-zalcitabine-zidovudine therapy for HIV-infected adults with CD4 cell counts between 50 and 350 per cubic millimeter. PISCES (SV14604) Study Group. *AIDS.* 1999;13(7):851–858.

45. Chatterton ML, Scott-Lennox J, Wu AW. Scott J. Quality of life and treatment satisfaction after the addition of lamivudine or lamivudine plus loviride to zidovudine-containing regimens in treatment-experienced patients with HIV infection. *Pharmacoeconomics.* 1999;15(Suppl 1):67–74.

46. Revicki DA, Swartz C, Wu AW, Haubrich R, Collier AC. Quality of life outcomes of saquinavir, zalcitabine and combination saquinavir plus zalcitabine therapy for adults with advanced HIV infection with CD4 counts between 50 and 300 cells/mm^3. Antiviral Therapy. 1999;4(1):35-44.

47. Casado A, Badia X, Consiglio E, et al. COMBINE Study Team. Health-related quality of life in HIV-infected naive patients treated with nelfinavir or nevirapine associated with ZDV/3TC (the COMBINE-QoL substudy). *HIV Clin Trials.* 2004;5(3):132–139.

48. Mukherjee, J, Wu Y, Odeshoo L, Kelleher T, et al. Atazanavir maintained patient utility and improved quality of life, comparing favorably to LPV/RTV: 24-week data from BMS 043. Ninth European AIDS Conference. Warsaw, Poland, October 25–29, 2003.

49. Spilker B, ed. *Quality of Life and Pharmacoeconomics in Clinical Trials.* 2nd ed. Philadelphia: Lippincott-Raven; 1995.

50. Nunnally JC. *Psychometric Theory.* 2nd ed. New York: Basic Books; 1978:229–246.

51. McDowell I, Newell C. *Measuring Health: A Guide to Rating Scales and Questionnaires.* 2nd ed. New York: Oxford University Press; 1996.

52. Jenkinson C, McGee H. *Health Status Measurement: A Brief But Critical Introduction.* Oxford: Radcliffe Medical Press; 1998.

53. Hays RD, Anderson R, Revicki DA. Psychometric evaluation and interpretation of health-related quality of life data. In: Shumaker SA, Berzon RA, eds. *The International Assessment of Health-Related Quality Of Life: Theory, Translation, Measurement and Analysis.* Oxford: Rapid Communications; 1995:103–114.

54. Lydick EG, Epstein RS. Clinical significance of quality of life data. In: Spilker B, ed. *Quality of Life and Pharmacoeconomics in Clinical Trials.* 2nd ed. Philadelphia: Lippincott-Raven; 1995:461–465.

55. Juniper EF, Guyatt GH, Willan A, Griffith LE. Determining a minimal important change in a disease-specific quality of life questionnaire. *J Clin Epidemiol.* 1994;47:81–87.

56. Jaeschke R, Singer J, Guyatt GH. Ascertaining the minimal clinically important difference. *Control Clin Trials.* 1989;10:407–415.

57. Bullinger M, Hasford J. Evaluating quality of life measures for clinical trials in Germany. Control Clin. Trials, 1991;12:91S–105S.

58. Hunt SM. Cross-cultural issues in the use of socio-medical indicators. HealthPolicy, 1986;6:149–158.

59. Hunt SM, McKenna S. Cross-cultural comparability of quality of life measures. *Br J Med Econ.* 1992;4:17–23.

60. Bullinger M, Anderson R, Cella D, Aaronson, N. Developing and evaluating cross-cultural instruments from minimum requirements to optimal models. *Qual Life Res.* 1993;2:451–459.

61. Hui C, Triandis HC. Measurement in cross-cultural psychology: a review and comparison of strategies. *Cross Cultural Psychol.*1985;16:131–152.

62. Aaronson NK. Assessing the quality of life of patients in cancer clinical trials. *Eur J Cancer.* 1992;28:1307–1310.

63. Jaeschke R, Guyatt GH, Keller J, et al. Interpreting changes in quality of life scores in N of 1 randomized trials. *Control Clin Trials.* 1991;12:226S–233S.

64. Hopwood P, Stephens RJ, Machin D. Approaches to the analysis of quality of life data: experiences gained from a Medical Research Council Lung Cancer Working Party palliative chemotherapy trial. *Qual Life Res.* 1994;3:339–352.

65. Zwinderman AH. The measurement of change of quality of life in clinical trials. *Stat Med.* 1990;9:931–942.

66. Schumacher M, Oschewski M, Schulen G. Assessment of quality of life in clinical trials. *Stat Med.* 1991;10:1915–1930.

67. Fairclough DL, Gelber RD. Quality of life: statistical issues and analysis. In: Spilker B, ed. *Quality of Life and Pharmacoeconomics in Clinical Trials.* 2nd ed. Philadelphia: Lippincott-Raven; 1995:427–435.

68. Crosby RD, Kolotkin RL, Williams GR. Defining clinically meaningful change in health-related quality of life. *J Clin Epidemiol.* 2003;56(5):395–407.

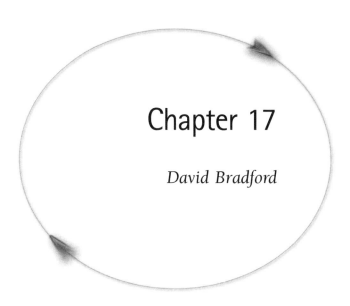

Chapter 17

David Bradford

Cost-Benefit Analysis in Health Services Research

Introduction

The health care arena is a sector of the economy where it is difficult to take market outcomes as normative. In the United States, while there may be many factors that move markets away from the ideal of perfect competition, typically the invisible hand of the economy is capable of efficiently allocating resources to individual markets. Masses of economists do not, for example, spend many hours estimating costs and benefits for the production of hamburgers in order to determine whether society should invest in a new franchise outlet. We let individuals choose whether to open a new outlet, safe in the knowledge that if the outlet is not socially optimal, then it (or another less efficient one) will be driven out of business. If it is socially efficient, then it will survive. This economic law of the jungle holds because individuals know what they are buying when they purchase a hamburger, costs of production are relatively predictable, and (most importantly) people pay for their consumption on the margin fully out of pocket.

In health care, however, frequently none of these conditions hold–particularly the latter. Consequently, when some agent in the market chooses to purchase a new technology, develop a new pharmaceutical product, or open a new clinic, this decision will not automatically be efficient. In fact, it is more often true that it will not be automatically efficient. We will discuss the reasons behind this briefly in the next section. For now, it is sufficient to note that since we cannot automatically assume that each health care resource allocation decision is efficient on average, then researchers must do the work of the market, and evaluate the efficiency of the decision in a research setting.

Until very recently, the method of cost-benefit analysis for these questions has been largely eschewed in favor of cost-effectiveness or cost-utility analysis. This is not due to any inherent advantage of these two methods. On the contrary, cost-effectiveness analysis is much more limited than cost-benefit analysis in terms of the scope of what the two procedures can address. Briefly, cost-effectiveness analysis typically involves estimating the costs in dollars of some intervention or investment and dividing those costs by the outcome obtained (see Chapters 13 and 14). For example, when considering the cost-effectiveness of beta-blocker therapy following a myocardial infarction, a typical cost effectiveness analysis will calculate the ratio of costs of beta-blocker therapy (direct costs of the drug plus any indirect costs attributable to the therapy) over the average number of recurrent myocardial infarctions within one year that are prevented (using the results of a clinical study). This ratio will be compared to a similar ratio for some other therapy (e.g., aspirin only therapy), and whichever intervention has the lower ratio will be judged best from all options studied. (For more details on the cost-effectiveness method, see the relevant chapter elsewhere in this volume.)

However, it should be apparent that such cost-effectiveness studies are strictly limited, in at least three ways: (1) the analysis ignores many other benefits from beta-blocker therapy, such as reduced incidents of angina, reduced severity of those myocardial infractions that do occur, reduced mortality, etc.; (2) the analysis assumes that some treatment is going to be applied—that is, it is strictly incorrect to compare the cost effectiveness of some therapy with the "cost effectiveness" of doing nothing, since that latter ratio must always equal zero; and (3) the analysis cannot readily compare the resource allocation for post-MI treatment to alternative uses of resources applied to, say, very low birth weight deliveries. Thus, cost-effectiveness is a tool that is very effective when one has already determined that some intervention is necessary, and the only remaining question is *how* to treat. But, cost-effectiveness is not appropriate when one wishes to ask *whether* some intervention should be undertaken. For that, one requires cost-benefit analysis. So in order to understand why cost-benefit analysis can provide this additional insight, we need to review what this type of analysis addresses.

This chapter will proceed by reviewing the economic principles that support cost-benefit analysis. Following this, we will discuss the general method of cost-benefit analysis, and then review briefly several traditional barriers to its use. Finally, we will present a discussion of the more recent advances in the field which have served to increase the acceptability and use of cost-benefit in health services research.

Chapter 17 • Cost-Benefit Analysis in Health Services Research **193**

Efficiency as an Economic Goal

The fundamental concepts of cost-benefit analysis can be easily illustrated using a simple model that would be familiar to most students of principles of economics. Figure 17-1 presents a graph of a simple (and heavily stylized) market for hamburgers. The downward sloping line represents the demand for hamburgers in our hypothetical market–where the demand (the maximum amount that consumers are willing and able to pay for each additional hamburger produced) also represents the marginal benefit to society from consuming hamburgers. This identity must hold true, since rational agents would only be willing to pay (out of pocket) as much for the last unit they consume as that unit brings them in value. Thus the area underneath the demand/marginal benefit curve for each unit represents the additional benefit that society receives from consuming that unit. The sum of these, up to the total number of hamburgers exchanged (H*) is the total benefit society receives from consuming hamburgers. Similarly, the upward sloping curve represents the supply, or marginal cost curve, and reflects the fact that since inputs (such as capital and labor) are not perfect substitutes, the opportunity cost of producing each additional unit will tend to rise as production increases. The area under the supply/marginal cost curve represents the additional opportunity cost in terms of resources that society must use up in order to produce each additional unit. Thus, the sum of these additional costs, up to the total number of hamburgers exchanged is equal to the total opportunity cost to society from the production of hamburgers.

In standard economic markets, such as those for hamburgers, supply and demand interact to assure that H* is actually produced, such that society retains as large an excess of total benefit over total

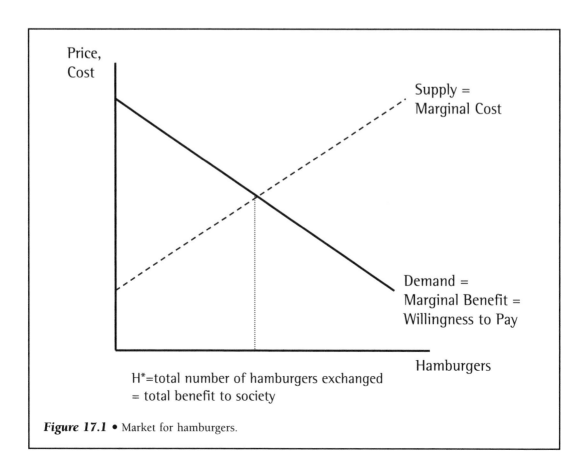

Figure 17.1 • Market for hamburgers.

opportunity costs. This excess benefit is known as surplus, and maximizing surplus is assured in competitive markets with no intervention. A cost-benefit analysis would simply amount to measuring the total benefit, measuring the total opportunity costs, and subtracting the two from each other to get a measure of surplus. As long as surplus is continuing to increase we would want to recommend continuing to increase production. Thus, one can see that cost-benefit analysis is, in principle, quite simple. The objective of cost-benefit analysis is simply to analytically measure the surplus represented in Figure 17.1 in order to assure that it is positive, and verify that any proposed increases in H would increase that surplus.

Of course, one would rarely consider conducting a cost-benefit analysis for the hamburger market. However, in health care such calculations are almost always required. The primary reason is that in health care, with widespread health insurance (such that very few people pay for care completely out of pocket), the market demand curve is not the true marginal benefit curve to society. As a result, the area under the demand curve will grossly over-state the true benefits from consumption, and health care markets will misallocate resources. Therefore, economists must step in to attempt to independently measure marginal benefits (in dollar terms), marginal costs, and thereby measure surplus. Measuring benefits satisfactorily has traditionally been the Achilles' heel of cost-benefit analysis.

Barriers to Benefit Measurement

Don Kenkel succinctly summarizes the major complaints that the clinical literature has with regard to cost-benefit analysis in an excellent *Journal of Health Economics* article from 1997.[1] The dominant complaint is that it is empirically difficult and even conceptually problematic to assign dollar values to the types of benefits (such as improvements in health, avoided deaths, gains in years of life) that are important in clinical research. It is certainly the case that early attempts at assigning dollar values to a year of life were weak, often resorting to measuring labor market productivity. However, there is now a large literature on valuing incremental changes in the risk of death, and even to valuing changes in mortality from investments in social programs (such as seat belt or airline safety regulation). This literature is summarized in an article written by Viscusi.[2] In addition, there is a growing body of work that utilizes contingent valuation methods to assess the value of improvements in health (such as reductions in the severity of angina pectoris or osteoarthritis). Thus, recent advances in the economic literature have significantly ameliorated the source of the empirical concern about cost-benefit analysis.

However, a conceptual problem still remains. Many clinicians appear to be unwilling to accept the ethical implications of assigning finite, measurable, values to human life. To this complaint, one need only conduct a simple thought experiment. Consider the spectacular wrecks that occasionally occur in auto racing. After the wreckage has come to a stop, it is not unusual to see the driver walking away from the accident unharmed. This raises the question of why it is that we have so many deaths on U.S. highways (where the highest observed speeds are much below that of the average auto race). The answer, of course, is that it is simply too expensive to build cars like those used in racing for daily use; while it is feasible, we do not observe any individuals actually demanding such cars. This means, of course, that individuals regularly trade off an increased risk of death for money (in the form of less expensive cars), implying that nearly no one in the U.S. driving public sets an infinite value on his or her own life. Once we can establish that the value each of us places on our own life is not infinite, then the conceptual objection collapses, and we are only left with wrestling with the empirical problems addressed above.

At this point, an aside is perhaps in order. As we have seen above, cost-benefit analysis has been greeted with skepticism largely because clinicians have been unwilling to agree that it is possible to set a dollar value on a year of human life.[3] Faced with this insurmountable obstacle to cost-benefit analysis, clinical researchers have most often resorted to cost-effectiveness analysis. However, frequently these cost-effectiveness analyses are conducted where there is no comparison option; that is, a single cost-effectiveness ratio is calculated (say, $75,000 per life year saved). Health services researchers are then at a loss. What does one do with the information that a new intervention is efficacious, but costs $75,000 to save one life. Is that good, or bad? When faced with this position, researchers resort to threshold values, most frequently asserting that $50,000 per life year saved is definitively "good" and that any gain between $50,000 and $100,000 per life year saved may be good, and that anything over $100,000 per life year saved is "bad."[4,5] This $50,000 per year value seems to have originated from a study of the costs of dialysis in Canada in the mid-1980s.[6] The astute reader will notice that such analyses are simply poorly-conducted cost-benefit analyses, where the dollar value of a year of life is arbitrarily set at $50,000 with certainty and $100,000 with some uncertainty. It is ironic that clinical researchers who so often decry the economists' practice of setting a dollar value on life as cold-hearted would resort to this tack since, as Hirth et al.[5] point out, economists would at least set the value of a year of life in the $400,000 range.

Recent Trends in Measuring Benefits from Health Interventions

There has been something of a rebirth in cost-benefit analysis since the early 1990s.[7–10] This rebirth is partly due to the increased attention that economists have paid to educating their clinical brethren about the superior theoretical and conceptual foundations of cost-benefit analysis compared to cost-effectiveness analysis. It is clear, for example, that if the perspective of the analysis is society, and if society is seeking to maximize welfare (social surplus), then cost-benefit analysis is the best (if not only) tool.[1]

However, the growth of cost-benefit analysis has also been spurred by the introduction of contingent valuation methods (primarily from the environmental economics literature), which seek to assign willingness to pay for non-market goods by the use of survey methods. A number of studies have demonstrated the generality of converting multi-dimensional preferences into a monetary index of willingness to pay (WTP) using "yes/no" or other dichotomous questions.[11] This method asks survey respondents whether they would be willing to pay a specific amount of money out of pocket for access to some treatment, technology, or health outcome. The dollar amount may be fixed, vary across a small number of values, or most recently, have unique values for each respondent.[12] Regression techniques are used to relate the "yes/no" answers to the dollar values asked and other characteristics of the respondents. The regression parameters can be used to predict willingness to pay for the good in question.

The applications of this technique are broad and growing. For example, WTP methods have been applied to health outcomes such as the value of reductions in the severity of angina pectoris attacks,[7,13] avoiding migraine headaches,[1] and avoiding post-operative nausea.[15] WTP has also been applied to health care services such as preventive medicine,[16] treatment for depression,[17] and to specific therapies.[18] It has only been in the past few years that clinical researchers have appeared to fully embrace the method of contingent valuation assessment of willingness to pay as a measure of the dollar value of benefits in health. In the first years of the 21st century, however, it would appear that cost-benefit analysis is well on its way to achieving the position of acceptance and even preference that it warrants, given its firm foundation in welfare theory.

How to Conduct a Cost-Benefit Analysis

The general approach for cost-benefit analysis is relatively straightforward, and is outlined in Gold et al.[3] Fundamentally, it involves identifying all opportunity costs associated with the intervention in question and comparing those to the dollar value of all benefits that accrue from the intervention. If the dollar values of the benefits exceed the opportunity costs, then the intervention improves social welfare and so should be adopted. Contrarily, if the opportunity costs exceed the benefits, then social surpluses will be reduced, and the intervention should not be adopted. The process involves four steps:

Step One: Identify All Opportunity Costs

- Identify the direct costs of potential treatment (e.g., costs of the intervention, costs of clinical personnel required to provide treatment, costs of supplies associated with treatment, etc.)
- Identify indirect costs associated with potential treatment and recovery (e.g., value of time lost from work or other activities associated with treatment, costs of ancillary health care that must be increased as a consequence of treatment, etc.)
- Identify expected costs associated with adverse outcomes from treatment (e.g., the dollar cost of treatment for some adverse event multiplied by the probabilities of the adverse event given treatment).

Step Two: Identify Clinical Benefits

- Identify changes in primary health indicators (e.g., reduction in heart attacks associated with treatment for hypertension)
- Identify changes in secondary health indicators (e.g., reduction in blood pressure associated with treatment for hypertension)
- Identify changes in level of morbidity
- Identify changes in life expectancy/mortality

Step Three: Identify Ancillary Benefits

- Implementing treatment under consideration may require fewer resources than current practice
- Treatment under consideration may save on non-health resources compared to current practice

Step Four: Value All Benefits

- Option 1: Assign dollar values to all clinical and ancillary benefits
- Option 2: Conduct willingness to pay study using identified benefits in the survey/instrument design.

This process is illustrated well in a study of the costs and benefits of hormone replacement therapy (HRT) by Zethraeus.[19] In this paper, the author seeks to determine whether HRT yields greater benefits to women in Sweden than the costs of providing the therapy. One interesting aspect of the analysis is that HRT has a wide range of benefits, in that it alleviates a range of menopausal symptoms, each of which would have to be valued separately if option one in step four above were followed. By implementing a WTP methodology, the author can avoid the need to capture each benefit of the therapy by hand, and can rather permit the women who are undergoing therapy to incorporate all benefits they receive into a single WTP measure.

Zethraeus administered a questionnaire to 104 women who utilize a single department of gynecology in a Swedish hospital. The questionnaire contained a contingent valuation question where all women were asked whether they would be willing to pay one of eight possible prices. The responses were used in a logit regression to calculate the mean willingness to pay for HRT among the women in the sample. The author found the mean WTP for HRT was approximately SEK 42,000 (approximately $5,314.00). The costs of the therapy can be easily calculated by measuring the price of the therapy, and the office visits required to monitor the therapy. These costs ranged between SEK 1,600 (approximately $202.00) and SEK 2,200 (approximately $278.00). Thus the value of the benefits were significantly more than the opportunity costs, implying the social welfare in Sweden is enhanced with the use of HRT.

A second example of a pharmacological cost-benefit study is found in Keith et al.[20] The authors conducted a study to compare the value of benefits from intranasal steroids for allergic rhinitis to the costs of the therapy. As in the previous example, given the range of benefits that are derived from alleviating the symptoms of allergic rhinitis, independently assessing clinical benefits and assigning distinct values to these benefits would be a daunting task. Consequently, a willingness to pay method was employed. The authors administered their instrument to 242 patients with positive diagnosis of allergic rhinitis (using a skin prick), who had been randomized into one of two treatment arms. Each patient was administered a willingness to pay instrument prior to the trial (where the hypothetical benefits were described). In this case, the patients were asked an open-ended question ("How much would you be willing to pay realistically each week to get rid of your ragweed hay fever and all the problems it brings?"). Patients were asked the same set of questions after completion of the clinical trial. Mean WTP was $12.95 per week. Opportunity costs of the therapy were tracked in the study, and included the dollar cost of the therapy, the number of unscheduled visits to the study physician and any other physician or clinic, and time off of work due to hay fever symptoms. Average per week opportunity costs were approximately $7.15. Again, since the dollar value of benefits exceeded the dollar value of costs, the therapy in question enhanced social welfare.

Summary

The health care sector is characterized by a large number of barriers which prevent normal market forces from acting to assure that resource allocations are efficient and maximize welfare. Consequently, it falls to economists and other health services researchers to calculate the net benefits of treatment and other resource allocation decisions. Since social welfare is theoretically based on the difference between the dollar value of total benefits and the dollar value of total opportunity costs, cost-benefit analysis is the gold standard method for health economic evaluations. Cost-benefit analysis involves measuring the value of benefits and subtracting from that the measured value of all costs (direct and indirect) of the decision in question. Since the 1990s, the most widely applied tool for assigning dollar values to benefits has been to estimate patient or social willingness to pay for the therapy in question. Such willingness to pay methods typically involve asking contingent valuation questions (either open ended "how much would you pay" questions, or dichotomous "would you pay a given amount" questions). The value of the willingness to pay method is that it allows the respondent to incorporate all dimensions of value into a single dollar amount. Additionally, the tools of contingent valuation estimation have become increasingly sophisticated. Given the growth of willingness to pay studies in recent years, the future of cost-benefit analysis in health economic and health services research is brighter than its past.

References

1. Kenkel, D. On valuing morbidity, cost-effectiveness analysis, and being rude. *J Health Econ.* 1997;16:749–757.

2. Viscusi, W, Magat W, Scharff R. Asymmetric assessments in valuing pharmaceutical risks. *Med Care.* 1996;34:DS34–47.

3. Gold M, et al. *Cost-effectiveness in Health and Medicine.* New York: Oxford University Press; 1996.

4. Ubel P, et al. What is the price of life and why doesn't it increase at the rate of inflation? *Arch Intern Med.* 2003;163:1637–1647.

5. Hirth R, et al. Willingness to pay for a quality-adjusted life year: in search of a standard. *Med Decision Making.* 2000;20:332–342.

6. Churchill, Lemon, Torrance. A cost-effectiveness analysis of continuous ambulatory peritoneal dialysis and hospital hemodialysis. *Medical Decision Making* 1984; 4: 489-500.

7. Johannesson M, Jonsson B, Borgquist L. Willingness to pay for antihypertensive therapy: results of a Swedish pilot study. *J Health Econ.* 1991;10:461–473.

8. Robinson, A. No prescription for despair. *Can Med Assoc J.* 1993;149:639–643.

9. O'Brien B, Gafni A. When do the "dollars" make sense? Toward a conceptual framework for contingent valuation studies in health care. *Med Decision Making* 1996;16:288–299.

10. Diener A, O'Brien B, Gafni A. Health care contingent valuation studies: a review and classification of the literature. *Health Econ.*1998;7:313–326.

11. van der Pol M, Ryan M, Donaldson C. Valuing food safety improvements using willingness to pay. *Appl Health Econ Health Policy.* 2003;2:99–107.

12. Bradford W, et al. Double-bounded dichotomous choice method to assess willingness to pay for telemedicine. Center for Health Care Research Working Paper. 2001. Charleston, SC: Medical University of South Carolina.

13. Chestnut L, et al. Measuring heart patients' willingness to pay for changes in angina symptoms. *Med Decision Making.* 1996;16:65–77.

14. Leslie, N. Insights into the pathogenesis of galactosemia. *Annu Rev Nutr.* 2003;23:59–80.

15. Tong, A. Clinical guidelines: can they be effective? *Nurs Times.* 2001;97:3–4.

16. Corso P, et al. Assessing preferences for prevention versus treatment using willingness to pay. *Med Decision Making.* 2002;22:S92–S101.

17. O'Brien W, VanEgeren L, Mumby P. Predicting health behaviors using measures of optimism and perceived risk. *Health Values: J Health Behav Ed Promotion.* 1995;19:21–28.

18. Ortega A, Dranitsaris G, Puodziunas A. A clinical and economic evaluation of red blood cell transfusions in patients receiving cancer chemotherapy. *Int J Technol Assess Health Care.* 1998;14:788–798.

19. Zethraeus, N. Willingness to pay for hormone replacement therapy. *Health Econ.* 1998;7:31–38.

20. Keith P, Haddon J, Birch S. A cost-benefit analysis using a willingness-to-pay questionnaire of intranasal budesonide for seasonal allergic rhinitis. *Ann Allergy Asthma Immunol.* 2000;84:55–62.

Appendix

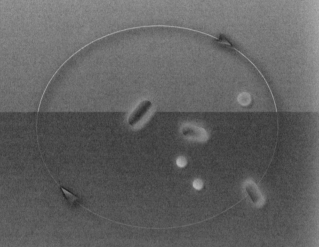

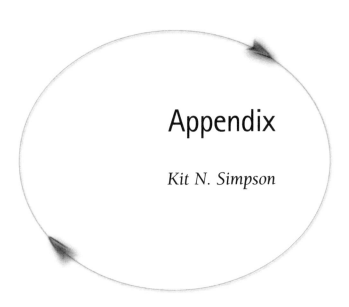

Appendix

Kit N. Simpson

Guide to Assessing Outcomes Research Studies

This text has attempted to give you the tools to understand the strengths and weaknesses of the many different methods that researchers use to compare the outcomes from different treatment approaches. However, you do not need every one of these tools every time you read a new study, so you need to be able to understand the individual contributions of each. Furthermore, while it is relatively easy to find the flaws in someone else's outcomes research design, it is close to impossible to design "flawless" outcomes research studies that are timely, and, therefore, may be used to inform discussions about clinical adoption or reimbursement policies before a new therapy is in common use.

The first thing to remember when you start reading an outcomes research study is that these are not clinical trials. Their purpose is different. They are not designed to measure efficacy but to help inform decision makers about either how efficacious therapies may be expected to work under real practice conditions, or how effective and/or costly new treatments are expected to be when they are used in routine practice.

Thus, these studies cannot be held to the same strict rules that guide the interpretation of clinical trial reports. However, just as there are good and bad clinical trials, so there are strong and weak outcomes research studies. The questions below may help you read outcomes research studies and judge how worthy they are of contributing to your store of evidence for and against the adoption of a new therapy. Read a new study with the following questions in mind:

What are the research objectives?

Which decisions are the authors trying to inform, given the study hypotheses:
• Better outcomes or quality of life with different treatments?
• Cost neutrality, cost savings, or "good value for the money" of a new treatment with a higher cost than currently available therapies?

Is the design and statistical approach appropriate?

• Have the authors controlled for selection bias?
• Have they maximized power to detect cost differences? Few clinical studies have enough power to detect statistically significant cost differences because costs usually have very large variances and skewed distributions.
• Have the authors transformed skewed data to fit the assumptions of their statistical approaches? Costs often need to be log-transformed to fit linear regression assumptions.
• Have the authors measured differences in quality of life for patients, or differences in how patients value the outcomes?
• Have the researchers used appropriate stochastic modeling approaches to capture the long-term impacts of cost and outcome differences which may be inferred from short-term clinical trial results?

How representative is the patient population, the practice setting, and the treatment process used?

• Is this strictly an efficacy study, or does it address effectiveness under real practice conditions, with real uncertainties in diagnosis and for patients with comorbidities?
• Is the practice setting in the study likely to be more or less costly than your own practice site?
• Are there study protocol effects that influence the costs or benefits reported? Which way would they affect costs? Outcomes?

Are there serious biases in the study that the authors have NOT tried to control for, or at least elucidate?

• Confounding by indication or other selection bias issues?
• Omitted quality of life measures?
• Cost weights that do not increase with increasing disease severity?

- Inadequate sample size to detect important difference in resource consumption (costs)?
- Flawed modeling assumptions?

Is this study simply more data in support of your current practice, or is it early evidence that a current policy or practice should be reconsidered or a new therapy adopted?

- Should you consider the new treatment for certain patients?
- Should you re-evaluate your standard protocol?
- Can you use this study to argue for a change that may improve quality of care, even if it also increases your drug budget?

Glossary

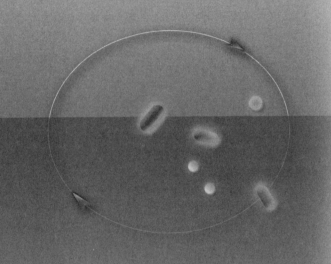

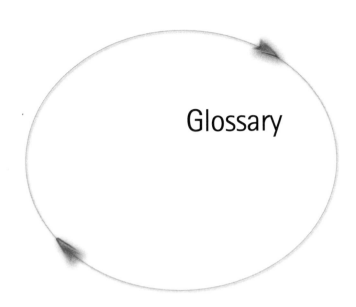

Glossary

Attributable Risk—A measure based on an absolute difference between incidence or risk estimates. It estimates the excess risk associated with the exposure of interest.

Absolute Risk Reduction—The difference in the risk of the outcome between subjects who have received one treatment from those who have received another. This measure provides the percentage of patients spared the adverse outcome as the result of receiving the experimental rather than the control therapy. Absolute risk reduction changes with a change in baseline risk.

Alpha—The probability of concluding that there is a difference between treatment groups when there really is not a difference between them; also known as the level of significance.

Alternative Hypothesis—The assumption that there is a difference between treatment effects.

Attrition Bias—Systematic differences between comparison groups in withdrawals or exclusions of participants from the results of a study. For example, participants may drop out of a study because of side effects of an intervention, and excluding these participants from the analysis could result in an overestimate of the effectiveness of the intervention, especially when the proportion dropping out varies by treatment group.

Beta—The probability of concluding that there is no difference between treatment groups when there really is a difference.

Bias—Systematic error that enters a clinical trial and distorts the data. Biases may be intentionally or unintentionally introduced into a clinical trial. Different types of biases include selection bias, recall bias, interviewer bias, etc. In statistical terms, bias refers to the situation where a sample is not representative of the population of interest.

Case-Control—An observational study in which subjects are selected on the basis of an outcome or disease of interest and are compared with respect to an exposure of interest.

Case Fatality Rates—The number of deaths from a specific disease or condition divided by the number of people with the disease or condition.

Case Report—A descriptive observational study in which some clinical outcome is reported with respect to person, place, time, or some other relevant variable.

Case Series—A descriptive observational study similar to a case report but that differs by examining more than one patient or subject.

Categorical Variable—A categorical variable (sometimes called a *nominal variable*) is one that has two or more categories, but there is no intrinsic ordering to the categories.

Chaining Estimates—A method for estimating standard gamble (or time trade-off) utility weights for a health state that only lasts for a short time. It requires a two-step procedure: first, by comparing the specific short duration health state to a lottery with the best and worst short duration health states, and, second, by comparing the worst health state assuming a lifetime duration with a lottery for death or perfect health.

Cohort Study—An observational study in which a group or groups of individuals are defined on the basis of an exposure to a suspected risk factor for a disease and then compared with respect to that disease.

Confidence Interval—An estimate of the range within which the true but unmeasured treatment effect lies in the larger population of interest.

Confounding Variable—A characteristic or factor that is unequally distributed between the treatment and control groups and affects the outcome of interest.

Contingent Valuation Method—Seeks to assign willingness to pay values for nonmarket goods by the use of survey methods.

Continuous Data—Data that have constant and defined units of measurement. There is an equal distance between increments of measure. Continuous data can be further divided into interval or ratio data. The ratio scale has an absolute zero, whereas the interval scale has the zero point arbitrarily assigned.

Correlation Analysis—Measures the strength of the association between two or more variables.

Correlation Coefficient—The correlation coefficient measures the degree to which two paired data sets are related.

Cost-Benefit Analysis—A process that involves identifying all opportunity costs associated with an intervention and comparing those costs to the dollar value of all benefits that accrue from the intervention. This analysis is used to determine whether some intervention should be undertaken.

Cost-effectiveness Analysis—Technique used to compare the cost and consequences of treatment alternatives that have a common non-monetary outcome.

Cost-effectiveness Ratio—Measure of economic efficiency calculated by dividing the cost of treatment by a non-monetary outcome such as years of life saved or cases prevented

Crossover Design—Allows each participant to receive both available treatment alternatives at different time periods, separated by a wash-out period between the treatments.

Cross-sectional Study—Studies in which information about the exposure and disease or outcome is obtained at the same time.

Cumulative Incidence—The number of new cases of disease or outcome that develop in a population at risk over a specified period of time divided by the number of persons at risk for developing the disease or outcome over a specified period of time.

Cumulative Meta-Analysis—A meta-analysis in which studies are added one at a time in a specified order (e.g., according to date of publication or quality) and the results are summarized as each new study is added. In a graph of a cumulative meta-analysis, each horizontal line represents the summary of the results as each study is added, rather than the results of a single study.

Demand/Marginal Benefit Curve—The maximum amount that consumers are willing and able to pay for each additional unit of product produced. The area underneath the demand/marginal benefit curve for each unit represents the additional benefit that society receives from consuming that unit.

Dependent Variable—Outcome of interest in a study.

Detection Bias—Systematic difference between comparison groups in how outcomes are ascertained, diagnosed, or verified.

Direct Cost—Medical and nonmedical expenditure directly related to the detection, treatment, and prevention of disease.

Discounting—Technique used to adjust future costs and consequences to current dollars; used to account for the time value of money.

Double Blinding—Investigators, participants, and, frequently, the biostatisticians evaluating the endpoints are all kept unaware of the treatment assignment.

Ecologic Analysis—An analysis that uses group-level or ecologic data to predict the group rate of an outcome such as disease.

Ecologic Fallacy—Mistakenly concluding that just because an association exists between an exposure and a disease at the group level of an ecologic analysis it also exists at the individual level.

Ecologic Study—Studies that examine the relationship between a risk factor and disease, but use naturally occurring groups of people, instead of individuals, as the unit of analysis.

Effectiveness—Effects of a treatment under real-world, everyday practice conditions.

Efficacy—Effects of a treatment under the controlled conditions of a clinical trial; efficacy is typically greater than effectiveness.

Efficiency—Output or outcome is achieved at the lowest possible cost.

Endpoints—The measurements that allow for the study hypotheses to be tested: can either be quantitative or qualitative in nature.

Experimental Study—Studies in which an investigator controls the intervention and then assesses its effect

Fixed-Effects Model—A model that calculates a pooled effect estimate using the assumption that all observed variation between studies is caused by the play of chance. Studies are assumed to be measuring the same overall effect. An alternative model is the random-effects model.

Gauss-Markov Theorem—States that in a linear model in which the errors have expectation zero and are uncorrelated and have equal variances the best linear unbiased estimators of the coefficients are the least-squares estimators.

Health Status—A "functional capacity" or "a state of physiological and psychological functioning or well-being." The World Health Organization (WHO) has also defined it as "the state of health of an individual, group, or population measured against accepted standards."

Health Utility—The level of well-being experienced by an individual in a particular state of health, generally determined by the individual's relative preference for that state compared to reference health states. The health state may be described by a single descriptor or by using multiple attributes.

Health Utility Weight—A number between 0 and 1 that reflects the level of well-being of an individual in a particular health state. The health state may be described by a single descriptor or by using multiple attributes.

Health-Related Quality of Life —Health-related quality of life represents the patient's perceptions and subjective evaluation of the functional effects of an illness and its consequent therapy upon him or her. Conceptually, HRQL encompasses the domains of emotional/psychological, physical, social, and role-functioning as well as general well-being. Spiritual and economic perceptions are sometimes included in the assessment as well.

Heterogeneity—Used specifically, as statistical heterogeneity, to describe the degree of variation in the **effect estimates** from a set of studies. Also used to indicate the presence of variability among studies beyond the amount expected due solely to the play of chance.

Heteroscedasticity—Unequal variance in the regression errors.

Homogeneity—Used specifically to describe the effect estimates from a set of studies where they do not vary more than would be expected by chance.

Huber-White Standard Errors—Standard errors which have been adjusted for specified assumed-and-estimated correlations of error terms across observations.

I^2—A measure used to quantify heterogeneity. It describes the percentage of the variability in effect estimates that is due to heterogeneity rather than sampling error (chance). A value greater than 50% may be considered to represent substantial heterogeneity.

Incidence Density—The number of new cases of disease or outcome that develop in a population at risk over a specified period of time divided by the total person-time of observation. Person-time is the sum of the times that each person under observation remained free from disease or outcome.

Independent Variable—Intervention or treatment in a study.

Indirect Cost—Cost related to changes in productivity of an individual due to illness.

Informed Consent—A process of communication between the clinical investigator and patient that ensures the complete understanding of the randomized clinical trial (including risks, costs, and other treatment options), allowing the potential participant to make an informed decision as to whether or not they wish to participate.

Intangible Cost—Cost related to the effects of illness on quality of life and patient satisfaction; measure of pain and suffering attributable to illness.

Intent-to-Treat—Following randomization to a specific treatment group, each participant's data should be included in the primary analysis regardless of compliance with the protocol-specified intervention or follow-up requirements.

Interquartile Range—A measure of variability directly related to the median. It is described by the interval between the 25th and 75th percentile values. The interquartile range clearly defines where the middle 50% of measures occur and also indicates the spread of the data.

League Table—Ranking of treatment alternatives according to their cost-effectiveness or cost-utility ratios.

Linear Probability Model—Least squares regression with a dichotomous dependent variable.

Logistic Regression—An estimation technique similar to logit, except that the estimated coefficients are the odds ratios for the likelihood of the outcome represented by the dependent variable for someone with the characteristic represented by a variable relative to someone without that characteristic.

Logit—A nonlinear estimation technique that is frequently used for dichotomous dependent variables. The model assumes that the error term has a logistic distribution. The logit model allows the marginal effect of an explanatory variable to vary with the value or level of the explanatory variable.

Maximum Likelihood Estimation—An iterative estimation technique that chooses the set of model parameter estimates to make the probability of observing the data most likely.

Mean—The arithmetic average of individual data points (i.e., the sum of all data points divided by the number of data points). The mean is useful for describing continuous data.

Median—The value above which or below which half of the data points fall. It is the 50th percentile value of a distribution.

Meta-Analysis—Systematic review and pooling of results from similar studies to achieve an improved estimate of efficacy of effectiveness.

Mode—The most commonly obtained value in a distribution.

Mortality Rates—The number of deaths within a population over a specified period of time divided by the number of people in the population during that period of time.

Multicollinearity—In a multiple regression with more than one X variable, two or more X variables are collinear if they are nearly linear combinations of each other.

Multi-level Analysis—An analysis that extends beyond the study of individual epidemiological factors by simultaneously incorporating different levels of variables (i.e., individual, workplace, neighborhood, community, or region) that might also influence an individual's state of health.

Multinomial Logit—A nonlinear model appropriate for non-ordered categorical dependent variables.

Nominal Data—Data with named or numbered categories that have no implied rank or order. The categories of a nominal scale must be exhaustive and mutually exclusive.

Nonparametric Methods—Statistical methods used when the conditions for using a parametric test are not satisfied; also used for hypothesis testing of nominal and ordinal data.

Null Hypothesis—The assumption that there is no difference between treatment effects.

Numbers Needed to Treat—Indicates the number of patients who require treatment to prevent one event; computed by taking the inverse of the absolute risk reduction.

Observational Study—Study in which an investigator does not have control or influence over an intervention.

Odds Ratio—The odds of exposure in subjects with the disease divided by the odds of exposure in subjects without the disease.

Opportunity Cost—Whatever must be given up to obtain some item.

Ordered Logit—A nonlinear model appropriate for categorical dependent variables in which the categories have a specific ordering (e.g., greatest to least).

Ordinal Data—Data that have a limited number of possible categories but do have an implied order or rank. It is important to recognize that although the order or rank is understood, the distance between each increment of measure (i.e., categories) is not equal.

Parallel Design—Participants receive only one of the possible treatment alternatives.

Parametric Methods—Statistical methods used when the data are normally distributed and continuous.

Partial Blinding—Allows for the identification of study participants by their treatment group without revealing the treatment by name.

Patient Reported Outcomes—An umbrella term that includes outcomes data reported directly by patients. Such data may include global impressions, functional status, well-being, symptoms, health-related quality of life, satisfaction with treatment, and treatment adherence.

Performance Bias—Systematic differences between intervention groups in care provided apart from the intervention being evaluated. For example, if participants know they are in the control group, they may be more likely to use other forms of care. If care providers are aware of the group a particular participant is in, they might act differently. Blinding of study participants (both the recipients and providers of care) is used to protect against performance bias.

Period Prevalence—The number of new and existing cases of disease or outcome within a population at a specified time divided by the number of people within the population during a specified period of time.

Per-Protocol—Following randomization to a specific treatment group, each participant's data should only be included in the analysis when they are compliant with protocol procedures (so only the participants who took the intervention as assigned are evaluated).

Perspective (of a Study)—The point of view from which a study is designed and conducted; the perspective influences which cost and consequences are included in a study and how they are valued.

Phase I Studies—Conducted to assess the metabolism, absorption, toxicity, and pharmacological effects of a new drug in human studies.

Phase II Studies—Conducted to test the safety and efficacy in a larger population of patients who have the disease that the drug was designed to treat.

Phase III Studies—Conducted to compare the new treatment to the "gold standard" therapy currently used for the disease in question.

Phase IV Studies—Conducted following FDA approval of the drug or device and are considered postmarketing studies to gain further information on the treatment's effect within various populations to assess side effects, benefits, and optimal administration associated with long-term use.

Point Prevalence—The number of new and existing cases of disease or outcome within a population at a specified time divided by the number of people within the population at a specified time.

Population—Refers to the whole (i.e., the collection of all possible measurements that could be used to answer a study question).

Power—The ability to detect a difference if one exists; the probability of detecting a treatment effect if there truly is one.

Probit—An alternative to the logit model, the probit model assumes that the error term has a normal distribution instead of a logistic distribution.

Proportionate Mortality—The number of deaths attributed to a disease or condition within a specified time period divided by the total number of deaths in the population within a specified time period.

Proportions—A general measure that indicates the fraction of a population that has the disease or outcome of interest.

Prospective Cohort Study—A particular type of cohort study in which the study population is defined before the study begins and is followed for a period of time into the future.

Psuedo-R^2—Measure of goodness of fit for nonlinear estimation techniques such as logit or probit. The value ranges from 0 to 1, but calculated values may vary across programs because no single definition or formula exists.

Publication Bias—A bias caused by only a subset of all the relevant data being available. The publication of research can depend on the nature and direction of the study results. Studies in which an intervention is not found to be effective are sometimes not published. Because of this, systematic reviews that fail to include unpublished studies may overestimate the true effect of an intervention. In addition, a published report might present a biased set of results (e.g., only outcomes or sub-groups where a statistically significant difference was found).

P-value—The level of statistical significance. It is the probability of obtaining the observed difference between treatments in a study, if there is no "real" difference between treatments in the larger population of interest.

Quality-Adjusted Life Year—A universal health outcomes measure applicable to all individuals and all diseases, thereby enabling comparisons across diseases and across programs by combining gains/ losses in both quantity of life (mortality) and quality of life (morbidity) into a single measure.

R^2—The R-Square statistic measures how successful the fit is in explaining the variation of the data.

Random Effects Model—A statistical model in which both within-study sampling error (variance) and between-studies variation are included in the assessment of the uncertainty (confidence interval) of the results of a meta-analysis. When there is heterogeneity among the results of the included studies beyond chance, random-effects models will give wider confidence intervals than fixed-effect models.

Random Error—Error due to the play of chance. Confidence intervals and P-values allow for the existence of random error, but not systematic errors (bias).

Random Sample—Means that each member of the population who has primary hypercholesterolemia has an equal and independent chance of being included in the trial. The intent of randomization is to produce study groups that are homogeneous with respect to known and unknown risk factors, to remove selection bias, and to ensure that statistical tests will have valid significance levels.

Randomized Clinical Trial—A type of clinical investigation in which participants are assigned to different treatment groups by chance to ensure that characteristics of the groups are similar at the initiation of the protocol.

Range—The difference between the largest and the smallest values in the distribution.

Rates—A general measure that indicates how fast the disease or outcome is occurring in the population.

Regression Analysis—Is used to describe the relationship between two or more variables. In regression analysis, a linear equation is derived that best fits a set of data pairs (X_i, Y_i) represented as points on a scatter diagram. This equation can be used to predict values of the dependent variable (Y) for given values of the independent variable (X). The sample regression line estimates the population's regression line.

Relative Preference—The degree to which a person prefers one health state compared to reference health states such as perfect health or death.

Relative Risk—Compares the probability of an outcome among individuals who have a specified characteristic or who have been exposed to a risk factor to the probability of that outcome among individuals who lack the characteristic or who have not been exposed to a risk factor.

Relative Risk Reduction—Estimates the percentage of baseline risk that is removed as a result of therapy. This is the percent reduction in the experimental group event rate compared with the control group event rate.

Reliability—Addresses the extent to which the measurement obtained is reproducible; it is a measure of the randomness of the measurement process itself.

Research Hypothesis—The research hypothesis (i.e., alternative hypothesis), denoted as H_1, states that there is a difference between treatments with respect to the outcome of interest.

Residual—The residuals from a fitted model are defined as the differences between the response data and the fit to the response data at each predictor value.

Responsiveness—Relates to the instrument's ability to detect clinically meaningful changes over time when a patient improves or deteriorates.

Retrospective Cohort Study—A particular type of cohort study in which the study population is identified and assembled in the past on the basis of existing records and then followed forward in time.

Robust Standard Errors—Standard errors that are have been corrected for possible heteroscedasticity.

Sample—The subset of a population of interest that was studied.

Selection Bias—Systematic differences between comparison groups in prognosis or responsiveness to treatment. Random allocation with adequate concealment of allocation protects against selection bias. Other means of selecting who receives the intervention are more prone to bias because decisions may be related to prognosis or responsiveness to treatment.

Sensitivity Analysis—Technique used to account for uncertainty in economic models by relaxing assumptions and allowing values of key variables to change over some relevant range; if results of the model do not change, the model is said to be robust.

Single Blinding—Only the participants are kept unaware of the treatment assignment.

Standard Deviation—The measure of the average amount by which each observation a data set from the mean.

Standard Error of the Mean—A measure of the precision with which a single sample mean estimates the true, but unmeasured, mean in the larger population of interest.

Standard Gamble Lottery—A question that asks respondents to choose between either their current health state or a hypothetical health state that will be experienced with certainty or a lottery wherein they will either experience the best possible health state with probability p or the worst possible health state with probability (1-p).

Standardized Mortality Ratio—The number of observed deaths divided by the number of expected deaths. This ratio is used in the indirect method of age-adjustment in calculating mortality rates.

Stratum—A non-overlapping group.

Supply/Marginal Cost Curve—The maximum amount that sellers are willing and able to sell. The area under the supply/marginal cost curve represents the additional opportunity cost in terms of resources that society must use up in order to produce each additional unit.

Surplus—Situation in which quantity supplied is greater than quantity demanded.

Surrogate Endpoint—An endpoint that is used as a proxy for the "true" or final biological or clinical outcome.

Survival Analysis—Statistical procedure used when investigators are interested in evaluating the time-to-the-event-of-interest for the study subjects.

Time Trade-Off Question—A question that asks respondents to choose between their remaining life expectancy spent in either their current health state or a hypothetical health state or a shorter life expectancy spent in perfect health.

Type I Error (False-Positive Rate)—Occurs when one falsely rejects the null hypothesis when it is true (i.e., concluding there is a difference between populations when there really is not a difference).

Type II Error (False-Negative Rate)—Occurs when one fails to reject the null hypothesis when the alternative hypothesis is true (i.e., concluding that there is no difference between populations when in fact there really is a difference).

Utility—A quantitative expression of an individual's preference for, or desirability of, a particular state of health under conditions of uncertainty.

Validity—Describes how well a measurement tool or economic evaluation truly reflects the relevant treatment effect.

Visual Analogue Scale—A rating scale with values from 0, the worst possible health state, to 1, the best possible health state, that asks respondents to place their current health state or a hypothetical health state on the scale between the two extreme values.

Wald Test—A standard statistical test for hypothesis testing in logit, probit, and other nonlinear models. The process for the test in these applications is analogous to a t-test.

Willingness to Pay—Survey method in which participants are asked whether they would be willing to pay a specific amount of money out of pocket for access to some treatment, technology, or health outcome. The dollar amount may be fixed, vary across a small number of values, or have unique values for each respondent. Regression analysis is used to predict willingness to pay for the goods in question, using the survey responses.

Index

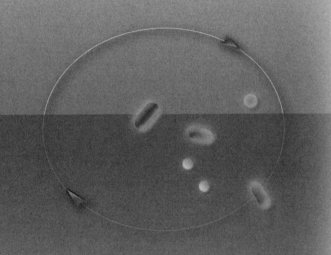

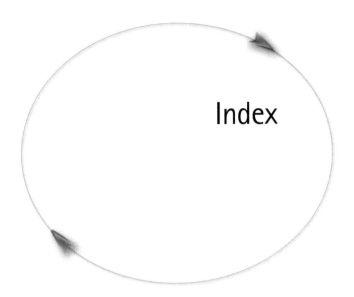

Index

A

Incremental cost effectiveness ratio (ICER), 134, 146, 148-49, 150, 151-52, 154-55
Incremental cost-utility ratio (ICUR), 152
Independence from irrelevant alternatives (IIA), 112
Independent study samples, 79
Independent variable (X), 24, 77, 95
Indirect age-adjustment, 20-21
Indirect costs, 143, 196
Individual-level studies, 25-26
Inferential statistics, 70
Influenza vaccination, 158
Informed consent, 51
Instantaneous risk, 9
Institutional review board (IRB), 53
Instrumental variable (IV), 89-90, 102
Insurance billing data, 120
Intangible costs, 143
Integrative decision model, 117
Intent-to-treat analyses, 51, 58, 62
Interaction term, 91, 100, 101, 110
Interferon-alpha2b, 153
Internal reliability, 180
Internal validity, 30
International Classification of Diseases, 9th edition (ICD9), 119
Interquartile range, 72
Interviewer/examiner objectivity, 39, 40
Intranasal steroids, 197
IRB. *See* Institutional review board
Item nonresponse, 186
IV. *See* Instrumental variable

J–K

Journal of Health Economics, 194
Kaplan-Meier curve, 80
Kenkel, Don, 194
Kitchen sink dilemma, 103
Kruskal-Wallis test, 79

L

Lamivudine, 128, 181, 182
Lead time bias, 123-24
Leflunomide, 11
Levin's Population Attributable Risk, 41
Linear probability model (LPM), 106, 108, 109, 111
Linear regression, 24, 25, 88-89, 90
Linkage variables, 119
Log viral load drop, 95, 96
Log-rank test, 80

Logistic regression, xiii, 89, 105-13
Logit model, 106-13
    extensions, 112
Loss to follow-up bias, 39, 40
Loviride, 182
LPM. *See* Linear probability model
Lung cancer screening, 123-24

M

Mann-Whitney U test, 79
Mantel-Haenszel chi, 79
Marginal effect, 110
Marker endpoints, 118, 119
Market price, 144
Markov model, 118, 124-26
    HIV disease, 126-28
MAUT. *See* Multiattribute utility theory
Maximum likelihood estimation (MLE), 107-8, 112-13
Maxwell, James, 6
MCID. *See* Minimal clinically important differences
Mean, 70, 71, 72
Measurement error, 102-3
Measurement scales, 77
Median, 70, 71, 72
Medicaid, 119, 139
Medical Outcomes Study (MOS)
    -HIV, 178, 181-84
    Short Form-36, 175, 177
Medicare, 120, 123, 154
Mental health summary (MHS), 177
Meta-analysis, xiii, 4, 57-64, 141
    example of, 62-63
    study eligibility, data search, 58-59, 60-61
MHS. *See* Mental health summary
Minimal clinically important differences (MCID), 187
Misclassification bias, 39
Missing data, 185-87
    imputation, 187
MLE. *See* Maximum likelihood estimation
Mode, 70, 71, 72
Model validation, 120
Modeling, 118-19, 128
Monte Carlo approach, 120
Mortality, 16-21, 49-50
Mortality rates, 16-17
MRI scan, 154
Multi-level analyses, 27
Multiattribute utility theory (MAUT), 166
Multicenter trials, 52-53
Multinomial logit model, 112